Taylor's Musculoskeletal Problems and Injuries

Taylor's Musculoskeletal Problems and Injuries
A Handbook

Robert B. Taylor, M.D.   Editor
Professor Emeritus
Department of Family Medicine
Oregon Health & Science University
  School of Medicine
Portland, Oregon

Associate Editors
Alan K. David, M.D.
Professor and Chairman
Department of Family and
  Community Medicine
Medical College of Wisconsin
Milwaukee, Wisconsin

Scott A. Fields, M.D.
Professor and Vice Chairman
Department of Family Medicine
Oregon Health & Science University
  School of Medicine
Portland, Oregon

D. Melessa Phillips, M.D.
Professor and Chairman
Department of Family Medicine
University of Mississippi
  School of Medicine
Jackson, Mississippi

Joseph E. Scherger, M.D., M.P.H.
Clinical Professor
Department of Family and
  Preventive Medicine
University of California,
  San Diego School of Medicine
San Diego, California

With 53 Illustrations

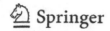 Springer

Robert B. Taylor, M.D.
Professor Emeritus
Department of Family Medicine
Oregon Health & Science University
  School of Medicine
Portland, OR 97239-3098, USA

Associate Editors

Alan K. David, M.D.
Professor and Chairman
Department of Family and
  Community Medicine
Medical College of Wisconsin
Milwaukee, WI 53226-0509, USA

D. Melessa Phillips, M.D.
Professor and Chairman
Department of Family Medicine
University of Mississippi School
  of Medicine
Jackson, MS 39216-4500, USA

Scott A. Fields, M.D.
Professor and Vice Chairman
Department of Family Medicine
Oregon Health & Science University
  School of Medicine
Portland, OR 97201-3098, USA

Joseph E. Scherger, M.D., M.P.H.
Clinical Professor
Department of Family and Preventive Medicine
University of California, San Diego
  School of Medicine
San Diego, California 92103-0801, USA

Library of Congress Control Number: 2005935915

ISBN-10: 0-387-29171-7
ISBN-13: 978-0387-29171-0

Preface

After more than a quarter century as a primary care educator, I am convinced that our graduates enter practice inadequately trained in the diagnosis and management of musculoskeletal problems and injuries. One reason for this perceived deficiency is the relatively short duration of primary care training—typically three years for family medicine, general internal medicine, and general pediatrics. During this time, there are just not enough months to teach all a clinician needs to know about diseases and trauma involving the musculoskeletal system. This inadequacy is compounded by the sometimes quirky nature of the problems: that is, for example, the increased risk of nonunion in a fracture of the carpal navicular (scaphoid) bone or the maneuver that can magically reduce a child's radial head subluxation.

The chapters in this book are from the edited reference book *Family Medicine: Principles and Practice*, 6th edition, which is widely used by family physicians in the United States and abroad. The publisher and I believe that, in addition to family physicians, the chapters in this book will also be useful to other clinicians providing broad-based care: general internists, general pediatricians, emergency physicians, nurse practitioners, and physician assistants. When compared to the large, comprehensive book, this volume will be preferred by some readers because of the physically smaller size and perhaps by the lower cost.

In selecting chapters to include in the book, I have included problems involving all areas of the skeleton and related musculature, in both children and adults. Athletic injuries are included because, after all, primary care clinicians manage most sports injuries. I have included a chapter on acute lacerations, which often accompany other types of injuries. In addition to sprains, strains, and fractures, there are chapters covering illnesses affecting the musculoskeletal system:

various types of arthritis, fibromyalgia, and the complex regional pain syndrome.

I hope you find this book useful in daily practice; comments are welcome.

Robert B. Taylor, M.D.
Portland, Oregon, USA

Clinical Practice Notice

Everyone involved with the preparation of this book has worked very hard to assure that information presented here is accurate and that it represents accepted clinical practices. These efforts include confirming that drug recommendations and dosages discussed in this text are in accordance with current practice at the time of publication. Nevertheless, therapeutic recommendations and dosage schedules change with reports of ongoing research, changes in government recommendations, reports of adverse drug reactions, and other new information.

A few recommendations and drug uses described herein have Food and Drug Administration (FDA) clearance for limited use in restricted settings. It is the responsibility of the clinician to determine the FDA status of any drug selection, drug dosage, or device recommended to patients.

The reader should check the package insert for each drug to determine any change in indications or dosage as well as for any precautions or warnings. This admonition is especially true when the drug considered is new or infrequently used by the clinician.

The use of the information in this book in a specific clinical setting or situation is the professional responsibility of the clinician. The authors, editors, or publisher are not responsible for errors, omissions, adverse effects, or any consequences arising from the use of information in this book, and make no warranty, expressed or implied, with respect to the completeness, timeliness, or accuracy of the book's contents.

Contents

Contributors

Allan V. Abbott, M.D., Professor of Family Medicine, Keck School of Medicine, University of Southern California, Los Angeles, California

Selected Injuries

Suraj A. Achar, M.D., Clinical Instructor of Family Medicine, University of California-San Diego School of Medicine, LaJolla, California

Musculoskeletal Problems of Children

Kenneth M. Bielak, M.D., Associate Professor of Family Medicine, University of Tennessee – Knoxville School of Medicine, Knoxville, Tennessee

Disorders of the Lower Extremity

Mark D. Bracker, M.D., Clinical Professor of Family and Preventive Medicine, University of California-San Diego School of Medicine, La Jolla, California

Musculoskeletal Problems of Children

Cora Collette Breuner, M.D., M.P.H., Department of Pediatrics, University of Washington Medical Center, Seattle, Washington

Athletic Injuries

Juan Carlos Buller, M.D., Staff Physician, San Diego Sports Medicine and Family Practice, San Diego, California

Musculoskeletal Problems of Children

Walter L. Calmbach, M.D., Associate Professor of Family and Community Medicine, Director of Sports Medicine Fellowship and South Texas Ambulatory Research Network (STARNET), University of Texas Health Science Center, San Antonio, Texas

Disorders of the Back and Neck

James F. Calvert Jr, M.D., Associate Professor of Family Medicine, Oregon Health & Science University School of Medicine, Portland; Cascades East Family Practice Residency Program, Klamath Falls, Oregon

Gout

Bryan J. Campbell, M.D., Assistant Professor of Family and Preventive Medicine, University of Utah School of Medicine, Salt Lake City, Utah

Care of Acute Lacerations

Douglas J. Campbell, M.D., Community Attending Physician, Good Samaritan Regional Family Practice Center, Yavapai Regional Medical Center, Prescott, Arizona

Care of Acute Lacerations

Joseph W. Gravel, Jr, M.D., Assistant Clinical Professor of Family Medicine and Community Health, Tufts University School of Medicine, Boston; Director, Tufts University Family Practice Residency Program, Malden, Massachusetts

Rheumatoid Arthritis and Related Disorders

Paula Cifuentes Henderson, M.D., Clinical Instructor of Family Medicine, University of California – Los Angeles School of Medicine, Los Angeles, California

Osteoporosis

Jeffrey G. Jones, M.D., M.P.H., Medical Director, St. Francis Traveler's Health Center, Indianapolis, Indiana

Selected Disorders of the Musculoskeletal System

Bradley E. Kocian, M.D., Sports Medicine Fellow, University of Tennessee -Knoxville Medical Center, Knoxville, Tennessee

Disorders of the Lower Extremity

Todd J. May, D.O., Lieutenant Commander, Medical Corps, United States Naval Hospital, Camp Pendleton, California

Musculoskeletal Problems of Children

Katherine E. Miller, M.D., Assistant Clinical Professor of Family Medicine and Community Health, Tufts University School of Medicine, Boston; Faculty, Tufts University Family Practice Residency Program, Malden, Massachusetts

Rheumatoid Arthritis and Related Disorders

Alicia D. Monroe, M.D., Associate Professor of Family Medicine, Brown Medical School, Providence; Memorial Hospital of Rhode Island, Pawtucket, Rhode Island

Osteoarthritis

John B. Murphy, M.D., Professor of Family Medicine, Brown Medical School, Providence, Rhode Island

Osteoarthritis

Doug Poplin, M.D., M.P.H., Medical Director, Saint Francis Occupational Health Center, Indianapolis, Indiana

Selected Disorders of the Musculoskeletal System

Ted C. Schaffer, M.D., Clinical Assistant Professor, Department of Family Medicine and Clinical Epidemiology, University of Pittsburgh School of Medicine; Director, UPMC – St. Margaret Hospital Family Practice Residency Program, Pittsburgh, Pennsylvania

Disorders of the Upper Extremity

Patricia A. Sereno, M.D., M.P.H., Assistant Clinical Professor of Family Medicine and Community Health, Tufts University School of Medicine, Boston; Hallmark Family Health Center, Malden, Massachusetts

Rheumatoid Arthritis and Related Disorders

Michael L. Tuggy, M.D., Clinical Assistant Professor of Family Medicine, University of Washington School of Medicine; Director, Swedish Family Medicine Residency Program, Seattle, Washington

Athletic Injuries

Richard P. Usatine, M.D., Professor of Clinical Family Medicine and Assistant Dean of Student Affairs, University of California – Los Angeles School of Medicine, Los Angeles, California

Osteoporosis

Wilma J. Wooten, M.D., M.P.H., Associate Clinical Professor of Family and Preventive Medicine, University of California-San Diego School of Medicine, La Jolla, California

Musculoskeletal Problems of Children

1
Disorders of the Back and Neck

Walter L. Calmbach

Disorders of the Back

Low back pain is a common and costly medical problem. The lifetime prevalence of low back pain is estimated to be 70% to 85%, and the point prevalence is approximately 30%.[1] Each year, 2% of all American workers have a compensable back injury, and 14% lose at least one workday due to low back pain.[2] Among chronic conditions, back problems are the most frequent cause for limitation of activity (work, housekeeping, school) among patients under 45 years of age.[3] Acute low back pain is the fifth most common reason for a visit to the physician, accounting for 2.8% of all physician visits.[4] And nonsurgical low back pain is the fourth most common admission diagnosis for patients over 65.[5] Although difficult to estimate, the direct medical costs due to back pain totaled $33.6 billion in 1994. Indirect costs (i.e., lost productivity and compensation) are estimated to be as high as $43 billion.[6] In most cases, low back pain is treated successfully with a conservative regimen, supplemented by selective use of neuroradiological imaging, and appropriate surgical intervention for a small minority of patients.[7]

Background
Epidemiology

Low back pain affects men and women equally, with the onset of symptoms between the ages of 30 and 50 years. It is the most common cause of work-related disability in people under 45 years of age, and is the most expensive cause of work-related disability.[8] Risk factors for the development of low back pain include heavy lifting and twisting, bodily vibration, obesity, and poor conditioning; however, low back pain is common even among patients without these risk factors.[1]

In cases of more severe back pain, occupational exposures are much more significant, including repetitive heavy lifting, pulling, or pushing, and exposures to industrial and vehicular vibrations. If even temporary work loss occurs, additional important risk factors include job dissatisfaction, supervisor ratings, and job environment (i.e., boring, repetitive tasks).[1] Factors associated with recurrence of low back pain include traumatic origin of first attack, sciatic pain, radiographic changes, alcohol abuse, specific job situations, and psychosocial stigmata.

Of patients with acute low back pain, only 1.5% develop sciatica (i.e., painful paresthesias and/or motor weakness in the distribution of a nerve root). However, the lifetime prevalence of sciatica is 40%, and sciatica afflicts 11% of patients with low back pain that lasts for more than two weeks.[9,10] Sciatica is associated with long-distance driving, truck driving, cigarette smoking, and repeated lifting in a twisted posture. It is most common in the fourth and fifth decades of life, and peaks in the fourth decade. Most patients with sciatica, even those with significant neurological abnormalities, recover without surgery.[11] Only 5% to 10% of patients with persistent sciatica require surgery.[5,12]

Despite the incidence and prevalence of low back pain and sciatica, the major factor responsible for its societal impact is disability.[12] The National Center for Health Statistics estimates that 5.2 million Americans are disabled with low back pain, of whom 2.6 million are permanently disabled.[13] Between 70% and 90% of the total costs due to low back pain are incurred by the 4% to 5% of patients with temporary or permanent disability.[12] Risk factors for disability due to low back pain include poor health habits, job dissatisfaction, less appealing work environments, poor ratings by supervisors, psychological disturbances, compensable injuries, and history of prior disability.[12] These same factors are associated with high failure rates for treatments of all types.

Natural History

Recovery from nonspecific low back pain is usually rapid. Approximately one third of patients are improved at one week, and two thirds at seven weeks. However, recurrences are common, affecting 40% of patients within six months. Thus, "acute low back pain" is increasingly perceived as a chronic medical problem with intermittent exacerbations.[14]

Low back pain may originate from many structures, including paravertebral musculature, ligaments, the annulus fibrosus, the spinal nerve roots, the facet joints, the vertebral periosteum, fascia, or blood vessels. The most common causes of back pain include musculoligamentous injuries, degenerative changes in the intervertebral discs and facet joints, spinal stenosis, and lumbar disc herniation.[14]

The natural history of herniated lumbar disc is usually quite favorable. Only about 10% of patients who present with sciatica have sufficient pain at six weeks that surgery is considered. Sequential magnetic resonance imaging (MRI) shows gradual regression of the herniated disc material over time, with partial or complete resolution in two thirds of patients by six months.[14] Acute disc herniation has changed little from its description in the classic article of Mixter and Barr: the annulus fibrosus begins to deteriorate by age 30, which leads to partial or complete herniation of the nucleus pulposus, causing irritation and compression of adjacent nerve roots.[5,13,16] Usually this herniation is in the posterolateral position, producing unilateral symptoms. Occasionally, the disc will herniate in the midline, and a large herniation in this location can cause bilateral symptoms. More than 95% of lumbar disc herniations occur at the L4–L5 or L5–S1 levels.[10] Involvement of the L5 nerve root results in weakness of the great toe extensors and dorsiflexors of the foot, and sensory loss at the dorsum of the foot and in the first web space. Involvement of the S1 nerve root results in a diminished ankle reflex, weakness of the plantar flexors, and sensory loss at the posterior calf and lateral foot.

Among patients who present with low back pain, 90% recover within six weeks with or without therapy.[17] Even in industrial settings, 75% of patients with symptoms of acute low back pain return to work within one month.[17] Only 2% to 3% of patients continue to have symptoms at six months, and only 1% at one year. However, symptoms of low back pain recur in approximately 60% of cases over the next two years.

Demographic characteristics such as age, gender, race, or ethnicity do not appear to influence the natural history of low back pain. Obesity, smoking, and occupation, however, are important influences.[18] Adults in the upper fifth quintile of height and weight are more likely to report low back pain lasting for two or more weeks.[9,18] Occupational factors that prolong or delay recovery from acute low back pain include heavier job requirements, job dissatisfaction, repetitious or boring jobs, poor employer evaluations, and noisy or unpleasant working conditions.[16] Psychosocial factors play an important role in the natural history of low back pain, modulating response to pain, and promoting illness behavior. The generally favorable natural history of acute low back pain is significantly influenced by a variety of medical and psychosocial factors that the practicing physician must be familiar with in order to counsel patients regarding prognosis and treatment.

Clinical Presentation

History

Low back pain is a symptom that has many causes. When approaching the patient with low back pain, the physician should consider three important issues. Is a systemic disease causing the pain? Is the patient experiencing social or psychosocial stresses that may amplify or prolong the pain? Does the patient have signs of neurological compromise that may require surgical evaluation?[14] Useful items on medical history include: age, fever, history of cancer, unexplained weight loss, injection drug use, chronic infection, duration of pain, presence of nighttime pain, response to previous therapy, whether pain is relieved by bed rest or the supine position, persistent adenopathy, steroid use, and previous history of tuberculosis.[14] Factors that aggravate or alleviate low back pain should also be elicited. Nonmechanical back pain is usually continuous, whereas mechanical back pain is aggravated by motion and relieved by rest. Low back pain that worsens with cough has traditionally been associated with disc herniation, although recent data indicate that mechanical low back pain also worsens with cough. The presence of leg weakness or leg paresthesias in a nerve root distribution is consistent with disc herniation. Bowel or bladder incontinence with or without saddle paresthesias suggests the cauda equina syndrome; this is a surgical emergency and requires immediate referral to a surgeon. Hip pain can mimic low back pain, and is often referred to the groin, the anterior thigh, or the knee, and is worsened with ambulation. Patients with osteoarthritis or degenerative joint disease report morning stiffness, which improves as the day progresses. Patients with spinal stenosis report symptoms suggestive of spinal claudication, that is, neurological symptoms in the legs that worsen with ambulation. Spinal claudication is differentiated from vascular claudication in that the symptoms of spinal claudication have a slower onset and slower resolution. A history of pain at rest, pain in the recumbent position, or pain at night suggests infection or tumor as a cause for low back pain. Osteoporosis is a consideration among postmenopausal women or women who have undergone oophorectomy. These patients report severe, localized, unrelenting pain after even "minor" trauma. Patients who present writhing in pain suggest the presence of an intra-abdominal process or vascular cause for the pain, such as abdominal aortic aneurysm.

Physical Examination

The initial examination is fairly detailed. With the patient standing and appropriately gowned, the examining physician notes the stance and gait, as well as the presence or absence of the normal curvature of the spine (e.g., thoracic kyphosis, lumbar lordosis, splinting to one side, scoliosis). The range of motion of the back is documented, including flexion, lateral bending, and rotation. Intact dorsiflexion and plantar flexion of the foot is determined by observing heel-walk and toe-walk. Intact knee extension is determined by observing the patient squat and rise, while keeping the back straight.

With the patient seated, a distracted straight-leg raising test is applied. With the hip flexed at 90 degrees, the flexed knee is brought to full extension. A positive straight-leg raising test reproduces the patient's paresthesias in the distribution of a nerve root at <60 degrees of knee extension. Sensation to light touch and pinprick are examined and motor strength of hip and knee flexors is tested. The deep tendon reflexes are tested [knee jerk (L4), ankle jerk (S1)] and long tract signs are elicited by applying Babinski's maneuver (Table 1.1).

With the patient in the supine position, the straight-leg raising test is repeated. With the hip and knee extended, the leg is raised (i.e., the

Table 1.1. **Motor, Sensory, and Deep Tendon Reflex Patterns Associated with Commonly Affected Nerve Roots**

Nerve root	Motor reflexes	Sensory reflexes	Deep tendon reflexes
C5	Deltoid	Lateral arm	Biceps jerk (C5,C6)
C6	Biceps, brachioradialis, wrist extensors	Lateral forearm	Brachioradialis
C7	Triceps, wrist flexors, MCP extensors	Middle of hand, middle finger	Triceps jerk
C8	MCP flexors	Medial forearm	—
T1	Abductors and adductors of fingers	Medial arm	—
L4	Quadriceps	Anterior thigh	Knee jerk
L5	Dorsiflex foot and great toe	Dorsum of foot	Hamstring reflex (L5, S1)
S1	Plantarflex foot	Lateral foot, posterior calf	Ankle jerk

MCP = metacarpophalangeal.

hip is flexed). A positive test reproduces the patient's paresthesias in the distribution of a nerve root. Isolated low back pain does not indicate a positive straight-leg raising test. The crossed straight-leg raising test (i.e., reproduction of the patient's symptoms by straight-leg raising of the contralateral leg) is very specific for acute disc herniation, and suggests a large central disc herniation. The examining physician should realize that the straight-leg raising test is sensitive but not specific, whereas the crossed straight-leg raising test is specific but not sensitive.[14] Hip range of motion is then tested, and pain radiation to the groin, anteromedial thigh, or knee is documented.

A more detailed examination may be necessary in selected patients. If significant pathology is suspected in a male patient, the cremasteric reflex is tested; i.e., application of a sharp stimulus at the proximal medial thigh should normally cause retraction of the ipsilateral scrotum. With the patient in the prone position, the femoral stretch test is applied. While the hip and knee are in extension, the knee is flexed, placing increased stretch on the femoral nerve, which includes elements from the L2, L3, and L4 nerve roots (i.e., the prone knee-bending test). The hamstring reflex is tested by striking the semitendinosus and semimembranosus tendons at the medial aspect of the popliteal fossa. The hamstring reflex involves both the L5 and S1 nerve roots. Thus, an absent or decreased hamstring reflex in the presence of a normal ankle jerk response (S1) implies involvement of the L5 nerve root (Table 1.1). Sensation in the area between the upper buttocks is tested, as well as the anal reflex and anal sphincter tone (S2, S3, S4).

The clinical diagnosis of acute disc herniation requires repeated physical examination demonstrating pain or paresthesias localized to a specific nerve root, with reproduction of pain on straight-leg raising tests, and muscle weakness in the nerve-appropriate root distribution.

Diagnosis

Radiology

Plain Radiographs. Plain radiographs are usually not helpful in diagnosing acute low back pain, because they cannot demonstrate soft tissue sprains and strains, or an acute herniated disc. However, plain radiographs are useful in ruling out conditions such as vertebral fracture, spondylolisthesis, spondylolysis, infection, tumor, or inflammatory spondyloarthropathy[5,19] (Fig. 1.1). In the absence of neurologic deficits, plain radiographs in the evaluation of low back pain should be reserved for patients over 50 years of age, patients with a temperature

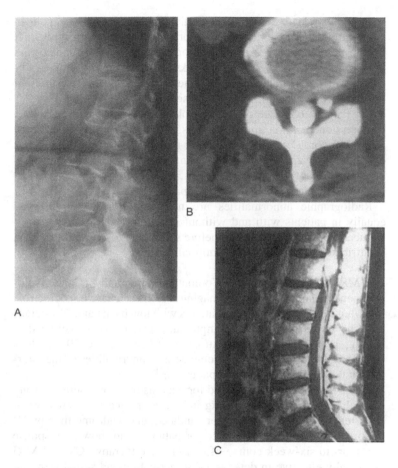

Fig. 1.1. Radiologic studies of the lumbar spine. (A) Plain radiograph demonstrating a compression fracture of the L2 vertebral body due to multiple myeloma. (B) CT scan demonstrating nucleus pulposus herniating posteriorly into the spinal canal. (C) MRI demonstrating an enhancing intramedullary metastatic lesion in the cauda equina at the L1 level.

>38°C, patients with anemia, a history of trauma, previous cancer, pain at rest, or unexplained weight loss, drug or alcohol abuse, steroid use, diabetes mellitus, or any other reason for immunosuppression.[20] For selected patients, initial plain radiographs of the spine in the early evaluation of acute low back pain should include anteroposterior and lateral views of the lumbar spine.[15] Oblique views are used to rule out

spondylolysis, particularly when evaluating acute low back pain in young athletic patients active in sports such as football, wrestling, gymnastics, diving, figure skating, or ballet.[21] If the patient's pain fails to improve after four to six weeks of conservative therapy, radiographs should be obtained; such patients may be at risk for vertebral infection, cancer, or inflammatory disease.[22]

For patients 65 years of age and older, diagnoses such as cancer, compression fracture, spinal stenosis, and aortic aneurysm become more common. Osteoporotic fracture may occur even in the absence of trauma. Because hormone replacement therapy and other medications may prevent further fractures, early radiography is recommended for older patients with back pain.[14]

Radiographic abnormalities are nonspecific and are observed equally in patients with and without symptoms of low back pain.[23] Clinical correlation is essential before symptoms of low back pain can be attributed to radiographic abnormalities.

CT, MRI, and Myelogram. Computed tomography (CT), myelogram, and magnetic resonance imaging (MRI) each have a specific role in evaluating a select subset of patients with low back pain. Physicians must be aware that many asymptomatic patients demonstrate disc bulging, protrusion, and even extrusion.[5,24] For example, 30% to 40% of CT scans and 64% of MRIs demonstrate abnormalities of the intervertebral disc in asymptomatic patients.[7,24]

CT or MRI should be reserved for patients in whom there is strong clinical suggestion of underlying infection or cancer, progressive or persistent neurological deficit, or cauda equina syndrome therapy.[5,14] CT or MRI should be considered for patients who show no response to a four- to six-week course of conservative therapy.[5] CT and MRI are equally effective in detecting disc herniation and spinal stenosis, but MRI is more sensitive in detecting infection, metastatic cancer, and neural tumors.[14] Myelography is useful in differentiating significant disc herniation from incidental disc bulging not responsible for the patient's signs or symptoms, but has largely been replaced by noninvasive techniques such as MRI or CT.[15] CT myelography is sometimes used in planning surgery.[14]

Ancillary Tests

Because plain radiographs are not highly sensitive for detection of early cancer or vertebral infection, tests such as erythrocyte sedimentation rate (ESR) and complete blood count (CBC) should be obtained for selected patients.[14,25]

Differential Diagnosis

Osteoarthritis

Osteoarthritis of the vertebral spine is common in later life, and is especially prevalent in the cervical and lumbar spine (also see Chapter 4). Typically, the pain of osteoarthritis of the spine is worse in the morning, increases with motion, but is relieved by rest. It is associated with morning stiffness, and a decreased range of motion of the spine in the absence of systemic symptoms. The severity of symptoms does not correlate well with radiographic findings, and patients with severe degenerative changes on plain radiographs may be asymptomatic, whereas patients with symptoms suggestive of osteoarthritis of the spine may have minimal radiologic findings. In some patients, extensive osteophytic changes may lead to compression of lumbar nerve roots or may even cause cauda equina syndrome.

Spinal Stenosis

Spinal stenosis is a common cause of back pain among older adults. Symptoms usually begin in the sixth decade, and over time the patient's posture becomes progressively flexed forward. The mean age of patients at the time of surgery for spinal stenosis is 55 years, with an average symptom duration of 4 years.[10] The symptoms of spinal stenosis are often diffuse because the disease is usually bilateral and involves several vertebrae. Pain, numbness, and tingling may occur in one or both legs. Pseudoclaudication is the classic symptom of spinal stenosis. Pseudoclaudication is differentiated from vascular claudication in that pseudoclaudication has a slower onset and a slower resolution of symptoms.[7]

Symptoms are usually relieved with flexion (e.g., sitting, pushing a grocery cart) and exacerbated by back extension. Plain radiographs often show osteophytes at several levels, but as mentioned earlier, caution must be used in ascribing back pain to these degenerative changes. CT or MRI may be used to confirm the diagnosis. Electromyography (EMG) or somatosensory evoked potentials may be used to differentiate the pain of spinal stenosis from peripheral neuropathy. The natural history of spinal stenosis is such that patients tend to remain stable or slowly worsen. Symptoms evolve gradually, but about 15% of patients improve over a period of about four years, 70% remain stable, and 15% experience worsening symptoms.[14] Nonoperative therapy for spinal stenosis includes leg strengthening and avoidance of alcohol to reduce the risk of falls, and physical activity such as walking or using an exercise bicycle is also recommended.[27] Decompressive laminectomy may be necessary for selected patients with spinal stenosis who have persistent severe pain. Although treatment for spinal stenosis must be individualized, recent reports suggest that patients treated surgically have better outcomes at four years than patients treated nonsurgically, even after adjusting for differences in baseline characteristics.[28] However, at four-year follow-up, 30% of patients still have severe pain and 10% have undergone reoperation.[28]

Osteoporosis

Osteoporosis is a common problem among seniors, affecting up to 25% of women over 65. Decreased bone mineral density in the vertebral body is associated with an increased risk for spinal compression fractures. In primary care settings, 4% of patients who present with acute low back pain have compression fractures as the cause.[14] Pain symptoms are worse with prolonged sitting or standing, and usually resolve over three to four months as compression fractures heal.[6] African-American and Mexican-American women have only one fourth as many compression fractures as European-American women.[5] Patients with compression fractures due to osteoporosis usually have no neurological complaints and do not suffer from neural compression. Plain radiographs document a loss of vertebral body height due to compression fractures. Laboratory tests are normal in primary osteoporosis, and any abnormalities should prompt a search for secondary causes of osteoporosis. The diagnosis of primary osteoporosis is made on clinical grounds, i.e., diffuse osteopenia, compression fractures, and normal laboratory findings.[29,30]

Neoplasia

Multiple myeloma is the most common primary malignancy of the vertebral spine. However, metastatic lesions are the most common cause of cancers of the spine, arising from breast, lung, prostate, thyroid, renal, or gastrointestinal tract primary tumors. Both Hodgkin's and non-Hodgkin's lymphomas frequently involve the vertebral spine. Because the primary site of the tumor is often overlooked, back pain is the presenting complaint for many cancers. In primary care settings, 0.7% of patients who present with low back pain have cancer as the cause.[10,25] Findings significantly associated with cancer as the cause of low back pain include age >50 years, previous history of cancer, pain lasting >1 month, failure to improve with conservative therapy, elevated ESR, and anemia.[25] Patients report a dull constant pain that is worse at night, and not relieved by rest or the recumbent position. Typical radiographic changes may be absent early in the course of vertebral body tumors. A technetium bone scan is usually positive due to increased blood flow and reactive bone formation; however, in multiple myeloma and metastatic thyroid cancer, the bone scan may be negative.[31] Greater diagnostic specificity and improved cost-effectiveness can be achieved by using a higher cut-off point for the ESR (e.g., >50 mm/hr) combined with either a bone scan followed by MRI as indicated, or MRI alone.[32] Symptomatic cancer of the lumbar spine is an ominous sign with a potential for devastating morbidity due to spinal cord injury.[33] Early recognition and treatment are essential if irreversible cord damage is to be avoided.

Posterior Facet Syndrome

The posterior facet syndrome is caused by degenerative changes in the posterior facet joints. These are true diarthrodial joints that sometimes develop degenerative joint changes visible on plain radiographs. Degenerative changes in the posterior facet joints cause a dull achy pain that radiates to the groin, hip, or thigh, and is worsened with twisting or hyperextension of the spine.[34] Steroid injection into the posterior facet joints to relieve presumed posterior facet joint pain is a popular procedure, but the placebo effect of injection in this area is significant and controlled studies have failed to demonstrate benefit from steroid injections.[35,36] The presence of degenerative changes in the facet joints on plain radiographs does not imply that the posterior facets are the cause of the patient's pain. Caution must be used in ascribing the patient's symptoms to these degenerative changes. Historically, the posterior facet syndrome was diagnosed by demonstrating pain relief after injection of local anesthetic into the posterior facet joints, but recent studies cast doubt on the validity of this procedure.[7,34] Several factors have been proposed to identify subjects who might benefit from lidocaine injection into lumbar facet joints: pain relieved in the supine position, age >65, and low back pain not worsened by coughing, hyperextension, forward flexion, rising from flexion, or extension-rotation.[37] However, a recent systematic review concluded that although facet joint injection provided some short-term relief, this benefit was not statistically significant; therefore, convincing evidence is lacking regarding the effects of facet joint injection therapy on low back pain.[38]

Ankylosing Spondylitis

Ankylosing spondylitis is a spondyloarthropathy most commonly affecting men under 40 years of age. Patients present with mild to moderate low back pain that is centered in the back and radiates to the posterior thighs. In its initial presentation, the symptoms are vague and the diagnosis is often overlooked. Pain symptoms are intermittent, but decreased range of motion in the spine remains constant. Early signs of ankylosing spondylitis include limitation of chest expansion, tenderness of the sternum, and decreased range of motion and flexion contractures at the hip. Inflammatory involvement of the knees or hips increases the likelihood of spondylitis.[39] The radiological hallmarks of ankylosing spondylitis include periarticular destructive changes, obliteration of the sacroiliac joints, development of syndesmophytes on the margins of the vertebral bodies, and bridging of these osteophytes by bone between vertebral bodies, the so-called bamboo spine. Laboratory analysis is negative for rheumatoid factor, but the ESR is elevated early in the course of the disease. Tests for human leukocyte antigen (HLA)-B27 are not recommended because as many as 6% of an unselected population test positive for this antigen.[15]

Visceral Diseases

Several visceral diseases may present with back pain as a chief symptom.[5] These include nephrolithiasis, endometriosis, and abdominal aortic aneurysm. Abdominal aortic aneurysm causes low back pain by compression of surrounding tissues or by extension or rupture of the aneurysm. Patients report dull steady back pain unrelated to activity, which radiates to the hips or thighs. Patients with an acute rupture or extension of the aneurysm report severe tearing pain, diaphoresis, or syncope, and demonstrate signs of circulatory shock.[29]

Cauda Equina Syndrome

The cauda equina syndrome is a rare condition caused by severe compression of the cauda equina, usually by a large midline disc herniation or a tumor.[14] The patient may report urinary retention with overflow incontinence, as well as bilateral sciatica, leg weakness, and sensory loss in a saddle distribution. Patients with these findings represent a true surgical emergency, and should be referred immediately for surgical treatment and decompression.

Psychosocial Factors

Psychological factors are frequently associated with complaints of low back pain, influencing both patient pain symptoms and therapeutic outcome.[40] Features that suggest psychological causes of low back pain include nonorganic signs and symptoms, dissociation between verbal and nonverbal pain behaviors, compensable cause of injury, joblessness, disability-seeking, depression, anxiety, requests for narcotics or other psychoactive drugs, and repeated failure of multiple treatments.[41] Prolonged back pain may be associated with failure of previous treatment, depression, or somatization.[14] Substance abuse, job dissatisfaction, pursuit of disability compensation and involvement in litigation are also associated with persistent unexplained symptoms.[8]

Management

Nonspecific Low Back Pain

For most patients, the best recommendation is rapid return to normal daily activities. However, patients should avoid heavy lifting, twisting, or bodily vibration in the acute phase.[14] A four- to six-week trial of conservative therapy is appropriate in the absence of cauda equina syndrome or a rapidly progressive neurological deficit (Table 1.2).

Bed Rest

Bed rest does not increase the speed of recovery from acute back pain, and sometimes delays recovery.[42,43] Symptomatic relief from back pain may benefit from one or two days of bed rest, but patients should be told that it is safe to get out of bed even if pain persists.[14]

Medications

Anti-inflammatories. Nonsteroidal anti-inflammatory drugs (NSAIDs) are effective for short-term symptomatic relief in patients with acute low back pain.[44] There does not seem to be a specific type of NSAID that is clearly more effective than others.[44] Therapy is titrated to provide pain relief at a minimal dose, and is continued for four to six weeks. NSAIDs should not be continued indefinitely, but rather prescribed for a specific period.[3]

Muscle Relaxants. Although evidence for the effectiveness of muscle relaxants is scant, the main value of muscle relaxants is less for muscle relaxation than for their sedative effect. Diazepam (Valium), cyclobenzaprine (Flexeril), and methocarbamol (Robaxin) are commonly used as muscle relaxants, and carisoprodol (Soma) has documented effectiveness.[3] Muscle relaxants should be prescribed in a time-limited fashion, usually less than two weeks. Muscle relaxants and narcotics are not recommended for patients who present with complaints of chronic low back pain (i.e., low back pain of greater than three months' duration).[5]

Unproven Treatments

Traction is not recommended for the treatment of acute low back pain.[45] No scientific evidence supports the efficacy of corsets or braces in the treatment of acute low back pain, and these treatments

Table 1.2. Nonoperative Treatment Considerations for Low Back Pain and Sciatica

Treatment	Acute low back pain	Acute sciatica	Subacute low back pain and leg pain	Chronic low back pain and leg pain
Bedrest	Avoid	Avoid	Avoid	Avoid, short-term for flare-ups only
NSAIDs	Symptomatic pain relief, time-limited	Symptomatic pain relief, time-limited	Selected cases if effective	Avoid long-term
Muscle relaxants	Optimal 1 week; maximum 2–4 weeks	Optimal 1 week; maximum 2–4 weeks	Selected cases if effective	Avoid long-term
Opioids	No	Optimal 1–3 days; maximum 2–3 weeks	Selected pre-surgical cases; avoid	Avoid
Antidepressants	No	No	Selected cases	Yes
Local injections	No	No	Selected cases as an adjunct	Flare-ups
Facet injections	No	No	No	Avoid; no long-term effect alone
Epidural corticosteroids	No	Yes	Flare-ups, if effective	Flare-ups only; avoid
Orthoses	Adjunctive	No	Adjunctive	Adjunctive
Cryotherapy (ice)	Adjunctive	Adjunctive	Flare-ups	Flare-ups; self-applied
Thermotherapy	Adjunctive	Adjunctive	Adjunctive	Flare-ups; self-applied

Traction	No	No	No	No
Joint manipulation	Not recommended for first 3–4 weeks	Not with neural signs	If effective; maximum 2–4 months	Flare-ups; time-contingent if effective
Joint mobilization	Yes, if effective	Yes, if effective	If effective; maximum 2–4 months	Flare-ups; time-contingent if effective
Soft tissue techniques (massage, myofascial release, mobilization)	Yes, if effective	Yes, if effective	If effective; maximum 2–4 months	Flare-ups; time-contingent if effective
McKenzie exercises	No	No	Flare-ups, if effective	Flare-ups, if effective
Dynamic lumbar stabilization	No	No	Yes	Yes
Back school	Yes	Yes	Yes	Yes
Functional restoration	No	No	Yes	Optimal 3–4 months; maximum 4–6 months
Pain clinic	No	No	No	Yes

NSAID = nonsteroidal antiinflammatory drug.
Source: Adapted from Wheeler,[41] with permission.

are not recommended.[5] Transcutaneous electrical nerve stimulation (TENS) is not effective in the treatment of low back pain.[46]

Exercise

Back exercises are not useful in the acute phase of low back pain, but are useful later for preventing recurrences.[14] Guidelines from the Agency for Health Care Policy and Research (AHCPR) stress aerobic exercise (e.g., walking, biking, swimming) especially during the first two weeks; continuing ordinary activities improves recovery and leads to less disability.[22] However, a recent systematic review concluded that specific back exercises do not improve clinical outcomes.[47] There is moderate evidence that flexion exercises are not effective in the treatment of acute low back pain, and strong evidence that extension exercises are not effective in the treatment of acute low back pain.

Spinal Manipulation

Clinical trials suggest that spinal manipulation has some efficacy.[48,49] Current recommendations are that patients should not be referred for spinal manipulation unless pain persists for more than three weeks because half of patients spontaneously improve during this time frame.[14]

Back School

A recent systematic review concluded that there is moderate evidence that back schools are not more effective than other treatments for acute low back pain.[50]

Acupuncture

A recent systematic qualitative review concluded that there is no evidence to show that acupuncture is more effective than no treatment, moderate evidence to show that acupuncture is not more effective than trigger point injection or TENS, and limited evidence to show that acupuncture is not more effective than placebo or sham procedure for the treatment of chronic low back pain.[51] Therefore, acupuncture is not recommended as a regular treatment for patients with low back pain.

Herniated Intervertebral Disc

Early treatment resembles that for nonspecific low back pain, outlined above. However, for patients with suspected lumbar disc herniation, the role of spinal manipulation is not clear. Narcotic analgesics may be necessary for pain relief for some patients with herniated interver-tebral disc, but these medications should be used in a time-limited (i.e., not symptom-limited) manner.[14] Epidural corticosteroid injec-tion may offer temporary symptomatic relief for some patients.[52] However, this invasive procedure offers no significant functional improvement, and does not reduce the need for surgery.[52] If neuro-pathic pain persists and/or neurological deficits progress, CT or MRI should be performed, and surgery should be considered.[14]

Surgery

Background. The rate of lumbar surgery in the United States is 40% higher than in most developed nations, and five times higher than in England and Scotland.[53] The lifetime prevalence of lumbar spine sur-gery ranges between 1% and 3%, and 2% to 3% of patients with low back pain may be surgical candidates on the basis of sciatica alone.[12] Surgery rates vary widely by geographical region in the United States and have risen dramatically in the last ten years.[54] Psychological fac-tors influence postsurgical outcomes more strongly than initial phys-ical examination or surgical findings. Prior to surgery, patients should be evaluated with standard pain indices, activities of daily living scales, and psychometric testing. Surgical results for treating sympto-matic lumbar disc herniation unresponsive to conservative therapy are excellent in well-selected patients.[55]

Indications. There is no evidence from clinical trials or cohort stud-ies that surgery is effective for patients who have low back pain unless they have sciatica, pseudoclaudication, or spondylolisthesis.[56] In the absence of cauda equina syndrome or progressive neurological deficit, patients with suspected lumbar disc herniation should be treated non-surgically for at least a month.[14] The primary benefit of discectomy is to provide more rapid relief of sciatica in patients who have failed to resolve with conservative management.[56] In well-selected patients, 75% have complete relief of sciatic symptoms after surgery and an additional 15% have partial relief. Patients with clear symptoms of radicular pain have the best surgical outcome, whereas those with the least evidence of radiculopathy have the poorest surgical outcome.[57] Relief of back pain itself is less consistent. Appropriate patient selec-tion is key to successful surgical outcome.

Options. Standard discectomy is the most common procedure used to relieve symptomatic disc herniation. A posterior longitudinal inci-sion is made over the involved disc space, a variable amount of bone is removed, the ligamentum flavum is incised, and herniated disc material is excised. This procedure allows adequate visualization and yields satisfactory results among 65% to 85% of patients.[11,58] Recent reports suggest that patients who undergo surgical therapy have greater improvement of their symptoms and greater functional recovery at four years than patients treated nonoperatively;[59] however, work status and disability status were similar between these two groups. Previous studies have shown that there is no clear benefit to surgery at ten-year follow-up.[11]

Microdiscectomy allows smaller incisions, little or no bony excision, and removal of disc material under magnification. This procedure has fewer complications, fewer unsuccessful outcomes, and permits faster recovery. However, rates of reoperation are significantly higher in patients initially treated with microdiscectomy, presumably due to missed disc fragments or operating at the wrong spinal level.[58] A recent systematic review concluded that the clinical outcomes for patients after microdiscectomy are comparable to those of standard discectomy.[56]

Percutaneous discectomy is an outpatient procedure performed under local anesthesia in which the surgeon uses an automated percutaneous cutting and suction probe to aspirate herniated disc material. This procedure results in lower rates of nerve injury, postoperative instability, infection, fibrosis, and chronic pain syndromes. However, patients undergoing percutaneous discectomy sustain unacceptably high rates of recurrent disc herniation. Only 29% of patients reported satisfactory results after percutaneous discectomy, whereas 80% of subjects were satisfied after microdiscectomy.[60] A recent systematic review concluded that only 10% to 15% of patients with herniated nucleus pulposus requiring surgery might be suitable candidates for percutaneous discectomy.[56] This procedure is not recommended for patients with previous back surgery, sequestered disc fragments, bony entrapment, or multiple herniated discs.[58,61]

For the time being, automated percutaneous discectomy and laser discectomy should be regarded as research techniques.[56] Arthroscopic discectomy is an emerging technique that shows promising results and effectiveness similar to that of standard discectomy.[62]

Chemonucleolysis is a procedure in which a proteolytic enzyme (chymopapain) is injected into the disc space to dissolve herniated disc material. A recent systematic review concluded that chemonucleolysis is effective for the treatment of patients with low back pain due to herniated nucleus pulposus, and is more effective than placebo.[56] However, chemonucleolysis showed consistently poorer results than standard discectomy. Approximately 30% of patients undergoing chemonucleolysis had further disc surgery within two years. Proponents of chemonucleolysis have suggested that it may be associated with lower costs, but readmission for a second procedure negates this putative advantage. Chemonucleolysis may be indicated for selected patients as an intermediate stage between conservative and surgical management.[56]

Complications. Complications of surgery on the lumbar spine are largely related to patient age, gender, diagnosis, and type of procedure.[63] Mortality rates increase substantially with age, but are <1% even among patients over 75 years of age. Mortality rates are higher for men, but morbidity rates and likelihood of discharge to a nursing home are significantly higher for women, particularly women over 75. With regard to underlying diagnosis, complications and duration of hospitalization are highest after surgery to correct spinal stenosis, degenerative changes, or instability, and are lowest for procedures to correct herniated disc. With regard to type of procedure, complications and duration of hospitalization are highest for procedures involving arthrodesis with or without laminectomy, followed by laminectomy alone or with discectomy, and are lowest for discectomy alone. Other surgical complications include thromboembolism (1.7%) and infection (2.9%).[5]

Summary

The physician's goal in treating patients with low back pain is to promote activity and early return to work. Although it is important to rule out significant pathology as the cause of low back pain, most patients can be reassured that symptoms are due to simple musculoligamentous injury.[14] Patients should be counseled that they will improve with time, usually quite quickly.

Bed rest is not recommended for the treatment of low back pain or sciatica; rather, a rapid return to normal activities is usually the best course.[14] Nonsteroidal anti-inflammatory drugs can be used in a time-limited way for symptomatic relief.[44] Back exercises are not useful for acute low back pain, but can help prevent recurrence of back pain and can be used to treat patients with chronic low back pain.[14] Work activities may be modified at first, but avoiding iatrogenic disability is key to successful management of acute low back pain.[5,41] Surgery should be reserved for patients with progressive neurological deficit or those who have sciatica or pseudoclaudication that persists after nonoperative therapy has failed.[14]

Chronic Low Back Pain

Chronic low back pain (i.e., pain persisting for more than three months) is a special problem that warrants careful consideration. Patients presenting with a history of chronic low back pain require an extensive diagnostic workup on at least one occasion, including in-depth history, physical examination, and the appropriate imaging techniques (plain radiographs, CT, or MRI).

Management of patients with chronic back pain should be aimed at restoring normal function.[47] Exercises may be useful in the treatment of chronic low back pain if they aim at improving return to normal daily activities and work.[47] A recent systematic review concluded that exercise therapy is as effective as physiotherapy (e.g., hot packs, massage, mobilization, short-wave diathermy, ultrasound, stretching, flexibility, electrotherapy) for patients with chronic low back pain.[47] And there is strong evidence that exercise is more effective than "usual care." Evidence is lacking about the effectiveness of flexion and extension exercises for patients with chronic low back pain.[47]

Although one literature synthesis cast doubt on the effectiveness of antidepressant therapy for chronic low back pain,[64] it is widely used and recommended.[14] Antidepressant therapy is useful for the one third of patients with chronic low back pain who also have depression. Tricyclic antidepressants may be more effective for treating pain in patients without depression than selective serotonin reuptake inhibitors.[65] However, narcotic analgesics are not recommended for patients with chronic low back pain.[14]

A recent systematic review concluded that there is moderate evidence that back schools have better short-term effects than other treatments for chronic low back pain, and moderate evidence that back schools in an occupational setting are more effective compared to placebo or "waiting list" controls.[50] Functional restoration programs combine intense physical therapy with cognitive-behavioral interventions and increasing levels of task-oriented rehabilitation and work simulation.[41] Patients with chronic low back pain may require referral to a multidisciplinary pain clinic for optimal management. Such clinics can offer cognitive-behavioral therapy, patient education classes, supervised exercise programs, and selective nerve blocks to facilitate return to normal function.[14] Complete relief of symptoms may be an unrealistic goal; instead, patients and physicians should try to optimize daily functioning.

Prevention

Prevention of low back injury and consequent disability is an important challenge in primary care. Pre-employment physical examination screening is not effective in reducing the occurrence of job-related low back pain. However, active aerobically fit individuals have fewer back injuries, miss fewer workdays, and report fewer back pain symptoms.[66] Evidence to support smoking cessation and weight loss as means of reducing the occurrence of low back pain is sparse, but these should be recommended for other health reasons.[66] Exercise programs that combine aerobic conditioning with specific strengthening of the back and legs can reduce the frequency of recurrence of low back pain.[44,66] The use of corsets and education about lifting technique are generally ineffective in preventing low back problems.[67,68] Ergonomic redesign of strenuous tasks may facilitate return to work and reduce chronic pain.[69]

Disorders of the Neck

Cervical Radiculopathy

Cervical radiculopathy is a common cause of neck pain, and can be caused by a herniated cervical disc, osteophytic changes, compressive pathology, or hypermobility of the cervical spine. The lifetime prevalence of neck and arm pain among adults may be as high as 51%. Risk factors associated with neck pain include heavy lifting, smoking, diving, working with vibrating heavy equipment, and possibly riding in cars.[70]

Cervical nerve roots exit the spine above the corresponding vertebral body (e.g., the C5 nerve root exits above C5). Therefore, disc herniation at the C4–C5 interspace causes symptoms in the distribution of C5.[71] Radicular symptoms may be caused by a "soft disc" (i.e., disc herniation) or by a "hard disc" (i.e., osteophyte formation and foraminal encroachment).[71] The most commonly involved interspaces are C5–6, C6–7, C4–5, C3–4, and C7–T1.[70]

The symptoms of cervical radiculopathy may be single or multiple, unilateral or bilateral, symmetrical or asymmetrical.[72] Acute cervical radiculopathy is commonly due to a tear of the annulus fibrosus with prolapse of the nucleus pulposus, and is usually the result of mild to moderate trauma. Subacute symptoms are usually due to long-standing spondylosis accompanied by mild trauma or overuse. The majority of patients with subacute cervical radiculopathy experience resolution of their symptoms within six weeks with rest and analgesics. Chronic radiculopathy is more common in middle age or old age, and patients present with complaints of neck or arm pain due to heavy labor or unaccustomed activity.[72–74]

Cervical radiculopathy rarely progresses to myelopathy, but as many as two thirds of patients treated conservatively report persistent symptoms. In severe cases of cervical radiculopathy in which motor function has been compromised, 98% of patients recover full motor function after decompressive laminectomy.[75]

Clinical Presentation

Among patients with cervical radiculopathy, sensory symptoms are much more prominent than motor changes. Typically, patients report proximal pain and distal paresthesias.[71] The fifth, sixth, and seventh nerve roots are most commonly affected. Referred pain caused by cervical disc herniation is usually vague, diffuse, and lacking in the sharp quality of radicular pain. Pain referred from a herniated cervical disc may present as pain in the neck, pain at the top of the shoulder, or pain around the scapula.[72]

On physical examination, radicular pain increases with certain maneuvers such as neck range of motion, Valsalva maneuver, cough, or sneeze. Active and passive neck range of motion is tested, examining flexion, rotation, and lateral bending. Spurling's maneuver is useful in assessing neck pain: the examining physician flexes the patient's neck, then rolls the neck into lateral bending, and finally extends the neck. The examiner then applies a compressive load to the vertex of the skull. This maneuver narrows the cervical foramina posterolaterally, and may reproduce the patient's radicular symptoms.

Diagnosis

The differential diagnosis of cervical nerve root pain includes cervical disc herniation, spinal canal tumor, trauma, degenerative changes, inflammatory disorders, congenital abnormalities, toxic and allergic conditions, hemorrhage, and musculoskeletal syndromes (e.g., thoracic outlet syndrome, shoulder pain).[71,75] In cases of cervical radiculopathy unresponsive to conservative therapy, or in the presence of progressive motor deficit, investigation of other pathologic processes is indicated. Plain radiographs are usually not helpful because abnormal radiographic findings are equally common among symptomatic and asymptomatic patients. CT scan, myelography, and MRI each have a specific role to play in the diagnosis of cervical radiculopathy.[73,74] CT scan is especially useful in delineating bony lesions, CT myelography can effectively demonstrate functional stenoses of the spinal canal, and MRI is an excellent noninvasive modality for demonstrating soft tissue abnormalities (e.g., herniated cervical disc, spinal cord derangement, extradural tumor).

Management

Immobilization. The purpose of neck immobilization is to reduce intervertebral motion which may cause compression, mechanical irritation, or stretching of the cervical nerve roots.[76] The soft cervical collar or the more rigid Philadelphia collar both hold the neck in slight flexion. The collar is useful in the acute setting, but prolonged use leads to deconditioning of the paracervical musculature. Therefore, the collar should be prescribed in a time-limited manner, and patients should be instructed to begin isometric neck exercises early in the course of therapy.

Bed Rest. Bed rest is another form of immobilization that modifies the patient's activities and eliminates the axial compression forces of gravity.[76] Holding the neck in slight flexion is accomplished by arranging two standard pillows in a V shape with the apex pointed cranially, then placing a third pillow across the apex. This arrangement provides mild cervical flexion, and internally rotates the shoulder girdle, thereby relieving traction on the cervical nerve roots.

Medications. Nonsteroidal anti-inflammatory drugs (NSAIDs) are particularly beneficial in relieving acute neck pain. However, side effects are common, and usually two or three medications must be tried before a beneficial result without unacceptable side effects is achieved. Muscle relaxants help relieve muscle spasm in some patients; alternatives include carisoprodol (Soma), methocarbamol (Robaxin), and diazepam (Valium). Narcotics may be useful in the acute setting, but should be prescribed in a strictly time-limited manner.[76] The physician should be alert to the possibility of addiction or abuse.

Physical Therapy. Moist heat (20 minutes, three times daily), ice packs (15 minutes, four times daily or even hourly), ultrasound therapy, and other modalities also help relieve the symptoms of cervical radiculopathy.[76]

Surgery. Surgical intervention is reserved for patients with cervical disc herniation confirmed by neuroradiologic imaging and radicular signs and symptoms that persist despite four to six weeks of conservative therapy.[71]

Cervical Myelopathy

The cause of pain in cervical myelopathy is not clearly understood but is presumed to be multifactorial, including vascular changes, cord hypoxia, changes in spinal canal diameter, and hypertrophic facets. Therefore, patients with cervical myelopathy present with a variable clinical picture. The usual course is one of increasing disability over several months, usually beginning with dysesthesias in the hands, followed by weakness or clumsiness in the hands, and eventually progressing to weakness in the lower extremities.[72]

Clinical Presentation

In cases of cervical myelopathy secondary to cervical spondylosis, symptoms are usually insidious in onset, often with short periods of worsening followed by long periods of relative stability.[77] Acute onset of symptoms or rapid deterioration may suggest a vascular etiology.[71] Unlike cervical radiculopathy, cervical myelopathy rarely presents with neck pain; instead, patients report an occipital headache that radiates anteriorly to the frontal area, is worse on waking, but improves through the day.[72] Patients also report deep aching pain and burning sensations in the hands, loss of hand dexterity, and vertebrobasilar insufficiency, presumably due to osteophytic changes in the cervical spine.[71,72]

On physical examination, patients demonstrate motor weakness and muscle wasting, particularly of the interosseous muscles of the hand. Lhermitte's sign is present in approximately 25% of patients, i.e., rapid flexion or extension of the neck causes a shocklike sensation in the trunk or limbs.[71] Deep tendon reflexes are variable. Involvement of the anterior horn cell causes hyporeflexia, whereas involvement of the corticospinal tracts causes hyperreflexia. The triceps jerk is the reflex most commonly lost, due to frequent involvement of the sixth nerve root (i.e., the C5–6 interspace). Almost all patients with cervical myelopathy show signs of muscular spasticity.

Diagnosis

Radiologic Diagnosis in Cervical Spondylosis. Intrathecal contrast-enhanced CT scan is a highly specific test that allows evaluation of the intradural contents and the disc margins, and helps differentiate an extradural defect due to disc herniation from that due to osteophytic changes.[73] MRI allows visualization of the cervical spine in both the sagittal and axial planes. Resolution with MRI is sharp enough to identify lesions of the spinal cord and differentiate disc herniation from spinal stenosis.[73] CT scan is preferred in evaluating osteophytes, foraminal encroachment, and other bony changes. CT and MRI complement each other, and their use should be individualized for each patient.[74] Clinical correlation of abnormal neuroradiologic findings is essential because degenerative changes of the cervical spine and cervical disc are common even among asymptomatic patients.[73,74]

Management

Conservative Therapy. Most patients with cervical myelopathy present with minor symptoms and demonstrate long periods of non-progressive disability. Therefore, these patients should initially be treated conservatively: rest with a soft cervical collar, physical therapy to promote range of motion, and judicious use of NSAIDs. However, only 30% to 50% of patients improve with conservative management. A recent multicenter study comparing the efficacy of surgery versus conservative management demonstrated broadly similar outcomes with regard to activities of daily living, symptom index, function, and patient satisfaction.[77]

Surgery. Early surgical decompression is appropriate for patients with cervical myelopathy who present with moderate or severe disability, or in the presence of rapid neurological deterioration.[78] Anterior decompression with fusion, posterior decompression, laminectomy, or laminoplasty is appropriate to particular clinical situations.[79] The best surgical prognosis is achieved by careful patient selection. Accurate diagnosis is essential, and patients with symptoms of relatively short duration have the best prognosis.[71] If surgery is considered, it should be performed early in the course of the disease, before cord damage becomes irreversible.

Surgical decompression is recommended for patients with severe or progressive symptoms; excellent or good outcomes can be expected for approximately 70% of these patients.[77]

Cervical Whiplash

Cervical whiplash is a valid clinical syndrome, with symptoms consistent with anatomic sites of injury, and a potential for significant impairment.[80] Whiplash injuries afflict more than 1 million people in the U.S. each year,[81] with an annual incidence of approximately 4 per 1000 population.[82] Symptoms in cervical whiplash injuries are due to soft tissue trauma, particularly musculoligamentous sprains and strains to the cervical spine. After a rear-end impact in a motor vehicle accident, the patient is accelerated forward and the lower cervical vertebrae are hyper extended, especially at the C5–6 interspace. This is followed by flexion of the upper cervical vertebrae, which is limited by the chin striking the chest. Hyperextension commonly causes an injury to the anterior longitudinal ligament of the cervical spine and other soft tissue injuries of the anterior neck including muscle tears, muscle hemorrhage, esophageal hemorrhage, or disc disruption. Muscles most commonly injured include the sternocleidomastoid, scalenus, and longus colli muscles.

Neck pain and headache are the cardinal features of whiplash injury.[83] Injury to the upper cervical segments may cause pain referred to the neck or the head and presents as neck pain or headache. Injury to the lower cervical segments may cause pain referred to shoulder and or arm. Patients may also develop visual disturbances, possibly due to vertebral, basilar, or other vascular injury, or injury to the cervical sympathetic chain.[81]

After acute injury most patients recover rapidly: 80% are asymptomatic by 12 months, 15% to 20% remain symptomatic after 12 months, and only 5% are severely affected.[83] However this last group of patients generates the greatest healthcare costs.

Clinical Presentation

On history, patients describe a typical rear-end impact motor vehicle accident with hyperextension of the neck followed by hyperflexion. Pain in the neck may be immediate or may be delayed hours or even days after the accident. Pain is usually felt at the base of the neck and increases over time. Patients report pain and decreased range of motion in the neck, which is worsened by motion or activity, as well as paresthesias or weakness in the upper extremities, dysphagia, or hoarseness.

Physical examination may be negative if the patient is seen within hours of the accident. Over time, however, patients develop tenderness in the cervical spine area, as well as decreased range of motion and muscle spasm. Neurological examination of the upper extremity should include assessment of motor function and grip strength, sensation, deep tendon reflexes, and range of motion (especially of the neck and shoulder).

Diagnosis

Findings on plain radiographs are usually minimal. Five views of the cervical spine should be obtained: anteroposterior, lateral, right and left obliques, and the odontoid view. Straightening of the cervical spine or loss of the normal cervical lordosis may be due to positioning in radiology, muscle spasm, or derangement of the skeletal alignment of the cervical spine. Radiographs should also be examined for soft tissue swelling anterior to the C3 vertebral body, which may indicate an occult fracture. Signs of pre-existing degenerative changes such as osteophytic changes, disc space narrowing, or narrowing of the cervical foramina are also common. Electromyography and nerve conduction velocity tests should be considered if paresthesias or radicular pain are present. Technetium bone scan is very sensitive in detecting occult injuries. However, whiplash injuries usually cause soft tissue injuries that are not demonstrable with most of these studies. For example, MRI of the brain and neck of patients within two days of whiplash injury shows no difference between subjects and controls.[84] Therefore, CT or MRI should be reserved for patients with neurological deficit, intense pain within minutes of injury, suspected spinal cord or disc damage, suspected fracture, or ligamentous injury.[81,82]

Management

Many patients recover within six months without any treatment. However, treatment may speed the recovery process and limit the amount of pain the patient experiences during recovery.[82]

Rest. Although rest in a soft cervical collar has been the traditional treatment for patients with whiplash injury, recent studies indicate that prolonged rest (i.e., two weeks or more) and/or excessive use of the soft cervical collar may be detrimental and actually slow the healing process.[85] Initially, patients should be treated with a brief period of rest and protection of the cervical spine, usually with a soft cervical collar for three or four days. The collar holds the neck in slight flexion; therefore, the widest part of the cervical collar should be worn posteriorly. The cervical collar is especially useful in alleviating pain if worn at night or when driving. If used during the day, it should be worn one or two hours and then removed for a similar period in order to preserve paracervical muscle conditioning. The soft cervical collar should not be used for more than a few days; early in the course of treatment, the patient should be encouraged to begin mobilization exercises for the neck.[81]

Medications. NSAIDs are effective in treating the pain and muscle spasm caused by whiplash injuries. Muscle relaxants are a useful adjunct, especially when used nightly, and should be prescribed in a time-limited manner. Narcotics are usually not indicated in the treatment of whiplash injuries.

Physical Therapy. A treatment protocol with proven success involves early active range of motion and strengthening exercises.[86] Patients are instructed to perform gentle rotational exercises ten times an hour as soon as symptoms allow within 96 hours of injury. Patients who comply with early active treatment protocols report significantly reduced pain and a significantly improved range of motion.

Physical modalities alleviate symptoms of pain and muscle spasm. Early in the course of whiplash injuries, heat modalities for 20 to 25 minutes, every three to four hours, are useful. However, excessive use of heat modalities can actually delay recovery. Later in the course of whiplash injury, usually two to three days after injury, cold therapy is indicated to decrease muscle spasm and pain. Range of motion exercises followed by isometric strengthening exercises should be initiated early in the therapy of whiplash injuries, even immediately after injury. Patients should be given specific instructions regarding neck exercises and daily activities. Patient education programs regarding exercises, daily activities, body mechanics, and the use of heat and cold modalities, are also helpful. The patient should be encouraged to remain functional in spite of pain or other symptoms. Any increase in pain following exercise should not be seen as a worsening of the injury. Prolonged physiotherapy should be avoided, because it reinforces the sick role for the patient.[81]

Multimodal treatments maximize success rates after cervical whiplash injury.[82] The goals of therapy are to restore normal function and promote early return to work. Physical therapy is used to reduce inappropriate pain behaviors, strengthen neck musculature, and wean patients off use of a soft cervical collar. Occupational therapy is used to facilitate the patient's return to normal functioning in the workplace. Neuropsychological counseling may be helpful for some patients.

Intra-Articular Corticosteroid Injection.   Intra-articular injection of corticosteroids is not effective therapy for pain in the cervical spine following whiplash injury.[87]

Prognosis

Most patients with whiplash injuries have negative diagnostic studies but improve, although slowly and irregularly. Patients benefit from a program of rest, immobilization, neck exercises, and return to function. At two-year follow-up, approximately 82% of patients with whiplash injury can expect to be symptom-free. Patients with persistent symptoms are older, have more signs of spondylosis on cervical radiographs, and probably sustained more severe initial injuries. Patients symptomatic at two-year follow-up initially reported more pain, a greater variety of pain symptoms, had higher rates of pretraumatic headache, and had more rapid onset of postinjury symptoms. Symptomatic and asymptomatic patients were similar with regard to gender, vocation, and psychological variables.[88] Some patients who sustain a whiplash injury never recover completely, probably due to a combination of the severity of the injury, underlying cervical abnormalities, and psychosocial factors.[81]

References

1. Anderson GBJ. The epidemiology of spinal disorders. In Frymoyer JW, ed. *The Adult Spine: Principles and Practice*. 2nd ed. Philadelphia: Lippincott-Raven, 1997;93–141.
2. Loeser JD, Volinn E. Epidemiology of low back pain. *Neurosurg Clin North Am.* 1991;2:713–18.
3. Deyo RA. Conservative therapy for low back pain. *JAMA.* 1983; 250(8):1057–62.
4. Hart LG, Deyo RA, Cherkin DC. Physician office visits for low back pain: frequency, clinical evaluation, and treatment patterns from a U.S. national survey. *Spine.* 1995;20:11–19.
5. Deyo RA, Loeser JD, Bigos SJ. Herniated lumbar inter-vertebral disc. *Ann Intern Med.* 1990;112:598–603.
6. Frymoyer JW, Durett CL. The economics of spinal disorders. In: Frymoyer JW, ed. *The Adult Spine: Principles and Practice*. 2nd ed. Philadelphia: Lippincott-Raven, 1997;143–50.
7. Frymoyer JW. Back pain and sciatica. *N Engl J Med.* 1988;318(5): 291–300.
8. Anderson GBJ. Epidemiologic features of chronic low back pain. *Lancet.* 1999;354:581–5.
9. Deyo RA, Tsui-Wu YJ. Descriptive epidemiology of low back pain and its related medical care in the United States. *Spine.* 1987;12:264–8.
10. Deyo RA, Rainville J, Kent DL. What can the history and physical examination tell us about low back pain? *JAMA.* 1992;268(6):760–5.
11. Weber H. Lumbar disc herniation: A controlled prospective study with ten years of observation. *Spine.* 1983;8(2):131–40.
12. Frymoyer JW, Cats-Baril WL. An overview of the incidences and costs of low back pain. *Orthop Clin North Am.* 1991;22(2):263–71.
13. National Center for Health Statistics. Prevalence of selected impairments. U.S., 1977, series 10, number 132. Hyattsville, MD. DHHS publication (PHS) 81–1562, 1981.
14. Deyo RA, Weinstein JN. Primary care: Low back pain. *N Engl J Med.* 2001;344(5):363–70.
15. Wipf JE, Deyo RA. Low back pain. *Med Clin North Am.* 1995; 79(2):231–46.
16. Mixter WJ, Barr JS. Rupture of inter-vertebral disc with involvement of the spinal canal. *N Engl J Med.* 1934;211(5):210–5.
17. Spitzer WO, LeBlanc FE, Dupuis M, et al. Scientific approach to the assessment and management of activity related spinal disorders. A monograph for clinicians. Report of the Quebec Task Force on Spinal Disorders. Spine 1987;12(suppl 1):S1–59.

18. Frymoyer JW, Nachemson A. Natural history of low back disorders. In: Frymoyer JW, ed. *The adult spine: Principles and practice.* New York: Raven Press, 1991;1537–50.

19. Modic MT, Ross JS. Magnetic resonance imaging in the evaluation of low back pain. *Orthop Clin North Am.* 1991;22(2):283–301.

20. Deyo RA, Diehl AK. Lumbar spine films in primary care: Current use and effects of selective ordering criteria. *J Gen Intern Med.* 1986;1:20–5.

21. Hensinger RN. Spondylolysis and spondylolisthesis in children and adolescents. *J Bone Joint Surg.* 1989;71A(7):1098–107.

22. Bigos S, Bowyer O, Braen G, et al. Acute low back problems in adults. Clinical practice guideline no. 14. Rockville, MD: Agency for Health Care Policy and Research, December 1994. (AHCPR publication no. 95-0642.)

23. Frymoyer JW, Newberg A, Pope MH, Wilder DG, Clements J, MacPherson B. Spine radiographs in patients with low back pain: An epidemiological study in men. *J Bone Joint Surg.* 1984;66A(7):1048–55.

24. Jensen MC, Brant-Zawadzki MN, Obuchowski N, Modic MT, Malkasian D, Ross JS. Magnetic resonance imaging in people without back pain. *N Engl J Med.* 1994;331(2):69–73.

25. Deyo RA, Diehl AK. Cancer as a cause of back pain: Frequency, clinical presentation, and diagnostic strategies. *J Gen Intern Med.* 1988;3:230–8.

26. Garfin SR, Herkowitz HN, Mirkovic S. Spinal stenosis. *Inst Course Lect.* 2000;49:361–74.

27. Hilibrand AS, Rand N. Degenerative lumbar stenosis: Diagnosis and management. *J Am Acad Orthop Surg.* 1999;7:239–49.

28. Atlas SJ, Keller RB, Robson D, Deyo RA, Singer DE. Surgical and non-surgical management of lumbar spinal stenosis: Four-year outcomes from the Maine Lumbar Spine Study. *Spine.* 2000;25(5):556–62.

29. McCowin PR, Borenstein D, Wiesel SW. The current approach to the medical diagnosis of low back pain. *Orthop Clin North Am.* 1991;22(2): 315–25.

30. Barth RW, Lane JM. Osteoporosis. *Orthop Clin North Am.* 1988; 19(4):845–58.

31. Bates DW, Reuler JB. Back pain and epidural spinal cord compression. *J Gen Intern Med.* 1988;3:191–7.

32. Joines JD, McNutt RA, Carey TS, Deyo RA, Rouhani R. Finding cancer in primary care outpatients with low back pain: A comparison of diagnostic strategies. *J Gen Intern Med.* 2001;16(1):14–23.

33. Perrin RG. Symptomatic spinal metastases. *Am Fam Physician.* 1989;39(5):165–72.

34. Jackson RP. The facet syndrome: Myth or reality? *Clin Orthop.* 1992;279:110–21.

35. Carette S, Marcoux S, Truchon R, et al. A controlled trial of corticosteroid injections into facet joints for chronic low back pain. *N Engl J Med.* 1991;325(14):1002–7.

36. Lilius G, Laasonen EM, Myllynen P, Harilainen A, Gronlund G. Lumbar facet joint syndrome: A randomized clinical trial. *J Bone Joint Surg.* 1989;71B(4):681–4.

37. Revel M, Poiraudeau S, Auleley GR, et al. Capacity of the clinical picture to characterize low back pain relieved by facet joint anesthesia.

Proposed criteria to identify patients with painful facet joints. *Spine*. 1998;23(18):1972–7.

38. Nelemans PJ, deBie RA, deVet HC, Sturmans F. Injection therapy for subacute and chronic benign low back pain. *Spine*. 2001;26(5):501–15.

39. Gran JT. An epidemiological survey of the signs and symptoms of ankylosing spondylitis. *Clin Rheumatol*. 1985;4:161–9.

40. Frymoyer JW, Rosen JC, Clements J, Pope MH. Psychologic factors in low back pain disability. *Clin Orthop*. 1985;195:178–84.

41. Wheeler AH. Diagnosis and management of low back pain and sciatica. *Am Fam Physician*. 1995;52(5):1333–41.

42. Waddell G, Feder G, Lewis M. Systematic reviews of bedrest and advice to stay active for acute low back pain. *Br J Gen Pract*. 1997;47:647–52.

43. Malmivaara A, Hakkinen U, Aro T et al. The treatment of acute low back pain—bedrest, exercises, or ordinary activity? *N Engl J Med*. 1995; 332:351–5.

44. van Tulder MW, Scholten RJ, Koes BW, Deyo RA. Nonsteroidal anti-inflammatory drugs for low back pain: A systematic review with the framework of the Cochrane Collaboration Back Review Group. *Spine*. 2000;25(19):2501–13.

45. Beurskens AJ, de Vet HC, Koke AJ, et al. Efficacy of traction for non-specific low back pain: 12-week and 16-month results of a randomized clinical trial. *Spine*. 1997;22:2756–62.

46. Deyo RA, Walsh NE, Martin DC, Schoenfeld LS, Ramamurthy S. A controlled trial of transcutaneous electrical nerve stimulation (TENS) and exercise for chronic low back pain. *N Engl J Med*. 1990;322(23):1627–34.

47. van Tulder M, Malmivaara A, Esmail R, Koes B. Exercise therapy for low back pain: A systematic review with the framework of the Cochrane Collaboration Back Review Group. *Spine*. 2000;25(21):2784–96.

48. Cherkin DC, Deyo RA, Battie M, Street J, Barlow W. A comparison of physical therapy, chiropractic manipulation, and provision of an educational booklet for the treatment of patients with low back pain. *N Engl J Med*. 1998;339:1021–9.

49. Anderson GBJ, Lucente T, Davis AM, Kappler RE, Lipton JA, Leurgans S. A comparison of osteopathic spinal manipulation with standard care for patients with low back pain. *N Engl J Med*. 1999;341:1426–31.

50. van Tulder MW, Esmail R, Bombardier C, Koes BW. Back schools for nonspecific low back pain (Cochrane Reivew). In: *The Cochrane Library*; issue 3. Oxford: Update Software, 1999.

51. van Tulder MW, Cherkin DC, Berman B, Lao L, Koes BW. The effectiveness of acupuncture in the management of acute and chronic low back pain. *Spine*. 1999;24(11):1113–23.

52. Carette S, Leclaire R, Marcoux S. Epidural corticosteroid injections for sciatica due to herniated nucleus pulposus. *N Engl J Med*. 1997; 336:1634–40.

53. Cherkin DC, Deyo RA, Loeser JD, Bush T, Waddell G. An international comparison of back surgery rates. *Spine*. 1994;19(11):1201–6.

54. Taylor VM, Deyo RA, Cherkin DC, Kreuter W. Low back pain hospitalization: recent U.S. trends and regional variations. *Spine*. 1994;19(11): 1207–13.

55. Hurme M, Alaranta H. Factors predicting the results of surgery for lumbar inter-vertebral disc herniation. *Spine.* 1987;12(9):933–8.
56. Gibson JNA, Grant IC, Waddell G. The Cochrane review of surgery for lumbar disc prolapse and degenerative lumbar spondylosis. *Spine.* 1999;24(17):1820–32.
57. Abramovitz JN, Neff SR. Lumbar disc surgery: Results of the prospective lumbar discectomy study. *Neurosurgery.* 1991;29(2):301–8.
58. Hoffman RM, Wheeler KJ, Deyo RA. Surgery for herniated lumbar discs: A literature synthesis. *J Gen Intern Med.* 1993;8:487–96.
59. Atlas SJ, Chang Y, Kamann E, Keller RB, Deyo RA, Singer DE. Long-term disability and return to work among patients who have a herniated disc: the effect of disability compensation. *J Bone Joint Surg.* 2000;82A(1):4–15.
60. Chatterjee S, Foy PM, Findaly GF. Report of a controlled clinical trial comparing automated percutaneous lumbar discectomy and microdiscectomy in the treatment of contained lumbar disc herniation. *Spine.* 1995;20:734–8.
61. Revel M, Payan C, Vallee C, et al. Automated percutaneous lumbar discectomy vs. chemonucleolysis in the treatment of sciatica. *Spine.* 1993; 18(1):1–7.
62. Hermantin FU, Peters T, Quartararo L, Kambin P. A prospective, randomized study comparing the results of open discectomy with those of video-assisted arthroscopic microdiscectomy. *J Bone Joint Surg.* 1999;81A:958–65.
63. Deyo RA, Cherkin DC, Loeser JD, Bigos SJ, Ciol MA. Morbidity and mortality in association with operations on the lumbar spine: The influence of age, diagnosis, and procedure. *J Bone Joint Surg.* 1992;74A(4): 536–43.
64. Turner JA, Denny MC. Do antidepressant medications relieve chronic low back pain? *J Fam Pract.* 1993;37(6):545–53.
65. Atkinson JH, Slater MA, Wahlgren DR, et al. *Pain.* 1999;83:137–45.
66. Lahad A, Malter AD, Berg AO, Deyo RA. The effectiveness of four interventions for the prevention of low back pain. *JAMA.* 1994;272(16): 1286–91.
67. Von Poppel MN, Koes BW, van der Ploeg T, Smid T, Bouter LM. Lumbar supports and education for the prevention of low back pain in industry. *JAMA.* 1998;279:1789–94.
68. Daltroy LH, Iversen MD, Larson MG, et al. A controlled trial of an educational program to prevent low back injuries. *N Engl J Med.* 1997;337:322–8.
69. Loisel P, Abenhaim L, Durand P, et al. A population-based, randomized clinical trial on back pain management. *Spine.* 1997;22(24):2911–18.
70. Kelsey JL, Githens PB, Walter SD, et al. An epidemiological study of acute prolapsed cervical intervertebral disc. *J Bone Joint Surg.* 1984;66A:907–14.
71. Clark CR. Degenerative conditions of the spine. In: Frymoyer JW, ed. *The Adult Spine: Principles and Practice.* New York: Raven Press, 1991;1145–64.
72. Lestini WF, Wiesel SW. The pathogenesis of cervical spondylosis. *Clin Orthop.* 1989;239:69–93.

73. Jahnke RW, Hart BL. Cervical stenosis, spondylosis, and herniated disc disease. *Radiol Clin North Am.* 1991;29(4):777–91.
74. Russell EJ. Cervical disc disease. *Radiology.* 1990;177(2):313–25.
75. Dillin W, Booth R, Cuckler J, Balderston R, Simeone F, Rothman R. Cervical radiculopathy: A review. *Spine.* 1986;11(10):988–91.
76. Murphy MJ, Lieponis JV. Non-operative treatment of cervical spine pain. In: Sherk HH, ed. *The Cervical Spine.* Philadelphia: Lippincott, 1989;670–7.
77. Sampath P, Bendebba M, Davis JD, Ducker TB. Outcome of patients treated for cervical myelopathy. *Spine.* 2000;25(6):670–6.
78. La Rocca H. Cervical spondylotic myelopathy: Natural history. *Spine.* 1988;13(7):854–5.
79. White AA 3rd, Panjabi MM. Biomechanical considerations in the surgical management of cervical spondylotic myelopathy. *Spine.* 1988;13(7): 856–69.
80. Hirsch SA, Hirsch PJ, Hiramoto H, Weiss A. Whiplash syndrome: Fact or fiction? *Orthop Clin North Am.* 1988;19(4):791–5.
81. Carette S. Whiplash injury and chronic neck pain. *N Engl J Med.* 1994;330(15):1083–4.
82. Eck JC, Hodges SD, Humphreys SC. Whiplash: A review of a commonly misunderstood injury. *Am J Med.* 2001;110(8):651–6.
83. Bogduk N, Teasell R. Whiplash: The evidence for an organic etiology. *Arch Neurol.* 2000;57(4):590–1.
84. Borchgrevink G, Smevik O, Haave I, et al. MRI of cerebrum and spinal column within 2 days after whiplash neck sprain injury. *Injury.* 1997;28:331–5.
85. Borchgrevink GE, Kaasa A, McDonagh D, et al. Acute treatment of whiplash neck sprain injuries. *Spine.* 1998;23:25–31.
86. Rosenfeld M, Gunnarsson R, Borenstein P. Early intervention in whiplash-associated disorders. A comparison of two treatment protocols. *Spine.* 2000;25:1782–7.
87. Barnsley L, Lord SM, Wallis BJ, Bogduk N. Lack of effect of intraarticular corticosteroids for chronic pain in the cervical zygapophyseal joints. *N Engl J Med.* 1994;330(15):1047–50.
88. Radanov BP, Sturzenegger M, DiStefano G. Long-term outcome after whiplash injury: a 2-year follow-up considering features of injury mechanism and somatic, radiologic, and psychosocial findings. *Medicine.* 1995;74(5):281–97.

2
Disorders of the Upper Extremity

Ted C. Schaffer

Because of the functional importance of the upper extremity to human activity, patients with injuries in this region frequently require diagnostic and therapeutic assistance from the family physician. A working knowledge of basic anatomy is helpful for establishing a differential diagnosis for upper extremity complaints. This chapter discusses common disorders in this region, but there are many unusual problems that may also present in an office situation.

Clavicle

The clavicle is the connecting strut that links the arm and shoulder with the axial skeleton. The clavicle is anchored medially by the sternoclavicular and costoclavicular ligaments, and the acromioclavicular and coracoclavicular ligaments anchor it to the scapula. A thorough examination of any shoulder injury should include palpation of the clavicle and evaluation of the acromioclavicular (AC) and the sternoclavicular (SC) joint motion.

Clavicular Fractures

Fractures of the clavicle are often due to a direct blow on the shoulder or occasionally to a fall on an outstretched arm.[1] They account for 5% of all fractures. Eighty percent of clavicular fractures occur in the middle third of the clavicle, especially at the junction of the middle and distal thirds.[2] Even when significant displacement or angulation is present, these fractures heal well with minimal intervention. A figure-of-eight sling or commercial clavicular strap, worn for three to four weeks by children and six weeks by an adult, provides effective immobilization and allows bony union.[1] The patient is advised that a permanent bump may become noticeable at the site of callus formation. Unless there is initial neurovascular injury, operative intervention or reduction is almost never required for fractures in the middle of the clavicle. Fractures of the distal third (15% of clavicular fractures) sometimes require surgery. Nondisplaced fractures that do not involve the AC joint heal without difficulty using the treatment outlined above. When a displaced or intra-articular fracture causes persistent pain, resection of the distal clavicle may be needed to alleviate discomfort. Fractures of the medial head of the clavicle (5% of fractures) or posterior dislocations at the sternoclavicular joint are fortunately rare. These injuries, caused by a direct blow to that region, may create a medical emergency by compressing the great vessels or compromising the airway. Immediate elevation of the impacted segment and urgent cardiothoracic or orthopedic consultation are recommended.

AC Joint Dislocations

Dislocations of the AC joint result from a direct fall onto the anterior shoulder. Management of this condition is determined by the extent of the dislocation. Specific treatment for this problem is covered in Chapter 9.

AC Joint Arthritis

With advancing age, there is an increased risk of AC joint arthritis, which may be interpreted as shoulder pain. Careful questioning frequently reveals a prior injury such as a grade I or II AC joint dislocation. Another potential source of injury is with extensive weight lifting. Degeneration of the cartilaginous meniscus may contribute to loss of AC joint integrity. On physical examination the patient is point tender over the AC joint. Forward flexion of the arm to 90 degrees followed by adduction of the shoulder, so the hand touches the contralateral shoulder (the crossed arm adduction test) compresses the AC joint and therefore reproduces the pain.

Initial treatment of AC joint arthritis includes rest, ice, and nonsteroidal anti-inflammatory drugs (NSAIDs). A corticosteroid injection into the AC joint using an anterior and superior approach may provide some benefit.[3] For cases unresponsive to conservative management, resection of the distal clavicle can alleviate persistent pain.

Scapula

Isolated injuries to the scapula are rare, but occasionally a direct blow over the involved area results in a fracture.[4] Because of the high impact involved, scapular fractures are frequently associated with other thoracic injuries such as rib fractures and pneumothorax. Treatment for fractures of the body of the scapula include immobilization with a sling until subsidence of pain within two to four weeks, followed by progressive exercises. If the acromion or glenoid is fractured, orthopedic referral is necessary because of potential implications to shoulder mobility and function.[4]

Shoulder

As the pivotal connection between the upper extremity and the axial skeleton, the shoulder is a frequent source of musculoskeletal problems. Its great range of motion is available only at some compromise to bony stability. Most shoulder stability is provided by the periarticular soft tissues. A careful physical examination attempts to identify which components are contributing to a specific problem. Disorders extrinsic to the shoulder may also cause referred pain to this area. An evaluation of the cervical spine should be included for any problem presenting as shoulder pain.

Functionally, the shoulder is composed of four joints: sternoclavicular, acromioclavicular, glenohumeral, and scapulothoracic articulation. The major joint is the glenohumeral joint, in which the humeral head is three times larger than the glenoid socket. A fibrocartilaginous glenoid labrum provides depth to the socket and adds stability. During overhead motion of the arm the humeral head is maintained in the socket by the four muscles of the rotator cuff. Originating from the scapula, these muscles maintain fixation of the humeral head and, based on their humeral insertion, assist in various arm motions. The supraspinatus assists in abduction and forward flexion, the infraspinatus and teres minor create external rotation, and the subscapularis causes internal rotation. Also vital for proper shoulder motion are the scapulothoracic muscles (rhomboid, trapezius, serratus anterior) and the deltoid.[5]

Traumatic Dislocation of the Shoulder
Anterior Dislocation

The major traumatic injury to the shoulder is dislocation of the humerus from the glenohumeral joint. About 95% of such dislocations are anterior,[6] caused by resisted force to the arm when the shoulder is abducted and externally rotated. Examination of this injury reveals a squaring of the shoulder, loss of the roundness of the deltoid muscle, prominence of the acromial edge, and an anterior mass, which is the humeral head. The arm is held in slight external rotation and abduction. Before reduction is attempted, a neurovascular examination assesses function of the anterior axillary nerve, which can be demonstrated as absent sensation over the deltoid region and loss of deltoid contraction. This injury, present with up to 30% of dislocations, is usually a transient neuropraxia that requires several weeks for neurological recovery.

If neurological evaluation of the dislocation reveals no other abnormality, immediate reduction is acceptable. A number of maneuvers have been described to relocate the shoulder.[4] Initial attempts emphasize gentle longitudinal traction on the arm while passive abduction and external rotation is performed. If there has been delay since the dislocation, narcotic analgesia is usually required to overcome muscle spasm. Most important with any maneuver is the caution that excessive torquing of the humerus must be avoided, as it may lead to brachial plexus injury or humeral fracture.

After relocation and repeat neurovascular evaluation, the patient is placed in a sling for a period of immobilization. A rehabilitation program is then instituted to strengthen the supportive musculature, restore motion, and prevent recurrent dislocation. Young patients, especially those under age 20, are at increased risk of recurrence (75–95%)[7] and require two to three weeks of immobilization before rehabilitation. For adolescents and young adults, failure to undergo and continue a satisfactory rehabilitation program is a frequent cause of recurrent dislocations. A shoulder stabilization procedure is often necessary for recurrent dislocators. In those over age 50, the risk of recurrent dislocation is much less (10%), but the increased risk of adhesive capsulitis and frozen shoulder requires that early shoulder motion be emphasized.[8] In this population an exercise program should be instituted after only one week of immobilization. Occasionally, especially in the elderly, there is an associated avulsion fracture of the greater tuberosity.

Subluxation

A more subtle problem is transient subluxation of the humerus, where the humeral head comes partially out of the anterior glenoid rim but then spontaneously reduces. Roentgenographic findings are negative, but the patient describes a transient "dead arm" feeling for several minutes after the initial injury. Later there may be persistent pain in the posterior shoulder due to a tear in the glenoid labrum. On physical examination a positive apprehension sign is noted, with pain when the shoulder is passively placed in abduction and externally rotated. A tear in the glenoid labrum may be a reason for chronic instability of the shoulder.

Those who experience a subluxation should undergo an aggressive rehabilitation program to prevent progression to dislocation. The advent of shoulder arthroscopy has improved the evaluation of patients with this problem.

Posterior Dislocation

Posterior dislocations comprise only 3% of shoulder dislocations but are missed on initial roentgenograms as often as 60% to 80% of the time.[6] They should be particularly suspected if there is a history of seizures, alcohol use, or electrical injury. On physical examination the arm is held in internal rotation, rather than the external rotation of anterior dislocation. Orthopedic consultation should be obtained if this injury is suspected.

Periarticular Shoulder Problems

Most shoulder problems involve the soft tissue periarticular shoulder structures rather than the glenohumeral joint. Because these supporting structures are vital to shoulder stability, a small injury to one component may cause significant problems in the motion and function of the shoulder. Classification is made difficult by the frequent overlap of these problems. At times one of the following specific periarticular shoulder problems is identified.

Rotator Cuff Injuries

Problems associated with the rotator cuff are the most frequent causes of shoulder problems. Impingement occurs chiefly in the supraspinatus as it courses underneath the acromion and coracoacromial ligament. Although this injury is most common in young athletes who engage in throwing or racquet sports, impingement may occur in anyone involved with overhead work or repetitive upper extremity motion. Evaluation of impingement syndromes is discussed in Reference 35, Chapter 52.

As a result of chronic impingement, the rotator cuff may tear. Cuff tears are more common in middle-aged or elderly individuals, often due to a hypovascular supply of the supraspinatus tendon as it inserts on the humerus.[9] One hallmark of cuff tears is continuous pain, especially at night, which may radiate down the lateral humerus.

Examination of the patient with a rotator cuff injury reveals painful or limited active abduction (between 60 and 120 degrees), where the cuff comes in greatest contact with the overlying acromial arch.[9] With a significant cuff tear, the patient is frequently unable to hold the arm in 90 degrees of abduction. Atrophy may develop in the supraspinatus or infraspinatus muscles of the scapula. If a cuff tear is suspected, orthopedic referral with arthroscopy or magnetic resonance imaging (MRI) is indicated to delineate potential surgical cases. With any cuff injury an extensive rehabilitation program of three to six months is needed to gain full motion and strength.

Subacromial Bursitis

The subacromial bursa separates the deltoid muscle from the underlying rotator cuff. Irritation of adjacent structures, most commonly impingement of the rotator cuff, results in inflammatory bursitis. Often there is a history of overuse or trauma followed by pain and limited active motion. Aspiration of excessive bursal fluid followed by corticosteroid injection using a subacromial lateral or posterior approach can provide dramatic relief of this problem.[3] Adequate volume of injection [5 to 10 cc lidocaine (Xylocaine) plus corticosteroid] should be used to optimize injection results.

Calcific tendonitis, usually within the supraspinatus insertion, may cause an acute inflammatory reaction of the overlying subacromial bursa. Roentgenograms demonstrate a calcific deposit superior and lateral to the humerus. The severe pain can be relieved by needle aspiration of the calcific mass along with a lidocaine and corticosteroid injection of the bursa. Occasionally surgical excision of the calcific deposition is required.[10]

Bicipital Tendonitis and Rupture

The long head of the biceps tendon, which is palpable in the bicipital groove, may be irritated as it courses through the glenohumeral joint and below the supraspinatus tendon to its attachment at the superior sulcus of the glenoid. Isolated pain over the long head of the biceps tendon suggests this problem, although usually there is more diffuse tenderness involving the entire subacromial region. The short head of the biceps tendon attaches to the coracoid process and is rarely involved in inflammatory problems of the shoulder. In most cases rupture of the long head of the biceps tendon occurs as a result of advanced impingement in middle-aged or elderly patients. There is a sudden pop associated with a heavy isometric flexion of the arm such as lifting a heavy object with that arm. The patient experiences mild discomfort with ecchymosis in the upper arm and a palpable bulge of the biceps muscle mass. Because the short head remains intact, treatment is symptomatic as little functional loss occurs.[11] Surgical repair is a rare consideration. Rupture of the distal insertion of the biceps tendon can also occur, with pain in the antecubital region. In contrast to proximal long head tear, this injury does warrant surgical repair.[11]

Glenohumeral Disorders

As a non-weight-bearing area, the true glenohumeral joint is subject to less mechanical stress than the lower extremity. When arthritic changes occur, there may have been a prior local injury. Inflammatory arthritis, with erosive changes of the glenohumeral joint and joint effusion, may occur, especially with severe rheumatoid arthritis.[12] Treatment for any degenerative arthritis is primarily aimed at relief of pain and inflammation. Surgical intervention with joint replacement is possible, but functional results are not as satisfactory as with knee and hip joint replacement, and the major goal should be relief of pain.

Adhesive Capsulitis

A poorly understood entity, adhesive capsulitis (also termed frozen shoulder or periarthritis) is characterized by a progressive, painful restriction of shoulder motion. A primary frozen shoulder has no apparent initiating event, is more common in the nondominant shoulder of women ages 40 to 60, and is bilateral in 20% of cases.[13] When there is a secondary cause of shoulder stiffness, such as immobilization, cuff injury, or trauma, the prognosis may not be as good, with permanent loss of shoulder motion. Initial treatment for either kind includes NSAIDs, joint injection, and an aggressive physical therapy program. For refractory cases other management options include manipulation under anesthesia or shoulder arthroscopy to lyse adhesions and enhance shoulder motion.[14]

Osteonecrosis

Although less common than osteonecrosis (avascular necrosis) of the femoral head, osteonecrosis of the humeral head may be caused by a number of illnesses such as alcoholism, sickle cell disease, systemic lupus erythematosus, and long-term steroid use.[15] Bone scan or MRI may be used for early diagnosis, as radiographs do not show subchondral collapse and humeral head flattening until later in the disorder. Treatment includes rest, analgesics, physical therapy for motion, and in severe cases joint replacement.

Humerus

Proximal humeral fractures occur in elderly patients who fall on an outstretched arm, with the fracture line at the surgical neck of the humerus. Although these fractures are frequently impacted, 80% of proximal humeral fractures are nondisplaced.[4] Because brachial plexus injury is possible, neurovascular examination is important with special attention to the axillary nerve. If there is less than 1 cm displacement and less than 45 degrees angulation, treatment is nonoperative (Fig. 2.1). A shoulder immobilizer is provided for one to two weeks, after which a sling is worn for another two weeks.[16] The major complication of these fractures in the elderly is loss of joint mobility, and an early exercise program beginning during the second week is important to maximize shoulder function. Even with rehabilitation some loss of shoulder abduction can be expected.

When a fracture involves the greater or lesser tuberosity or is associated with a humeral head dislocation, there is greater risk of long-term sequelae due to rotator cuff malfunction, and orthopedic consultation should be obtained. With trauma to the humeral shaft, which occurs in young active patients, the integrity of the adjacent radial nerve should be tested.

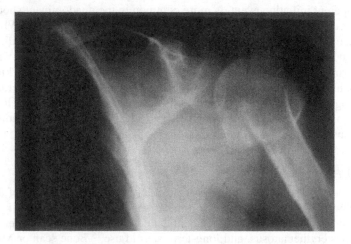

Fig. 2.1. This impacted humeral fracture in an elderly women is neither displaced nor severely angulated. It was successfully managed with an arm sling for a week followed by range of motion exercises and a course of physical therapy.

Elbow

Fractures of the Radial Head

One common uncomplicated elbow injury is a fracture of the proximal radial head. The history of a fall on an outstretched hand accompanies a patient who is reluctant to pronate the hand or to flex the elbow beyond 90 degrees.[17] Radiological examination of the radial head, especially on the lateral film, is important when the patient is unable to move the elbow through a complete range of motion. The only roentgenographic evidence for fracture may be a posterior fat pad sign, which occurs when blood that has entered the joint space displaces the fat pad posteriorly (Fig. 2.2).

Management of a nondisplaced radial head fracture emphasizes pain relief and, in adults, early mobilization. A sling and posterior elbow splint are worn for one to two weeks, after which range of motion (ROM) exercises are begun while the protective sling is worn for another week.[16] Follow-up of the patient is important for this seemingly trivial problem, as it may take several months for the patient to regain full elbow motion. If displacement of the head or severe angulation has occurred in a child, operative repair may be necessary because the radial head is necessary to provide adequate lengthening of the radius. In adults with radial head displacement or comminution, excision of the radial head is possible to permit adequate pain-free motion at the elbow.

Epicondylitis

Epicondylitis, a frequent elbow complaint, is caused by inflammation of the lateral or medial epicondyle. Although its diagnosis and treatment are covered in Reference 35, Chapter 52, the clinician must understand that epicondylitis is not always related to sports participation. Obtaining an accurate history usually identifies a causative action related to the patient's vocational or recreational activities.

Radial Head Subluxation

The most common elbow complaint in children, known as nurse-maid's elbow, occurs when sudden longitudinal traction on the wrist or arm causes the annular ligament to become partially entrapped in the radiohumeral joint. The child younger than four years old presents with a painful elbow held in pronation. Gentle rotation of the hand to a supinated position while pressure is applied over the radial head results in a palpable "click" as the radial head is reduced.[18] There is immediate pain relief with full use of the elbow. Radiographs are not

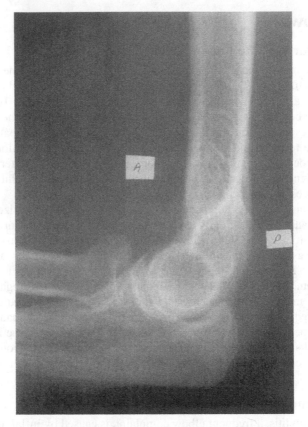

Fig. 2.2. Fat pad signs. A nondisplaced radial head fracture with both a posterior (P) and a prominent anterior (A) fat pad evident on this lateral view. The posterior fat pad is indicative of blood in the joint space from an occult fracture, displacing the fat from the joint space.

necessary; positioning for the radiograph may actually cause reduction of the subluxation. To prevent recurrence, parents and caregivers should be educated about the injury mechanism for this benign entity.

Olecranon Bursitis

Either a single traumatic blow to the elbow or repetitive microtrauma such as leaning on the elbow may result in swelling over the posterior aspect of the elbow. When there is marked inflammation, a septic bursitis is suspected. Treatment for a septic bursitis includes surgical drainage of the bursal fluid and intravenous antibiotics. *Staphylococcus aureus* is the most common infecting organism. For a simple noninfected bursitis, aspiration of clear, straw-colored fluid can be followed by a tight pressure dressing applied to prevent fluid reaccumulation.[19] When recurrent bursitis results in a thickened fibrotic mass, the only recourse may be surgical excision of the entire bursa.

Wrist

Fractures of the Distal Radius

Because of the close proximity to the radiocarpal joint, fractures of the distal radius are considered wrist injuries. In children the most common injury is the buckle, or torus, fracture, which occurs with a fall onto an outstretched hand. Radiographic findings may be subtle, with only a slight cortical disruption of the extra-articular radius seen on the lateral film (Fig. 2.3). Treatment is a short arm cast for three weeks; functional return is excellent.[20]

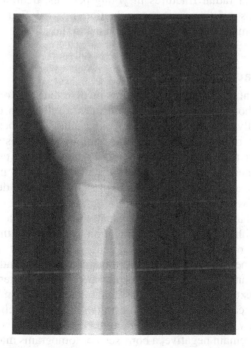

Fig. 2.3. Buckle (torus) fracture. A small cortical disruption is visible in the metaphysis of the distal radius.

When a child presents with a "sprained wrist," evaluation must be done carefully, as the growth plates are weaker than ligaments during this period of rapid growth. With normal roentgenograms and tenderness over the epiphyseal plate, a Salter I fracture is presumed, and a short arm cast is applied for two to three weeks.[20]

In adults the most common radial fracture is a Colles' fracture, which occurs when patients over age 50 fall onto an outstretched hand. The "silver fork" deformity is caused by dorsal displacement of the distal fragment. The ulnar styloid may also be fractured. Reduction of a Colles' fracture may be attempted, but the physician must be aware of potential complications of this fracture, including median or ulnar nerve compression, damage to the flexor or extensor tendons, and radioulnar joint arthritis.

Nondisplaced distal radial fractures that are nonarticular can usually be treated with cast immobilization for six weeks in adults. Low-impact intra-articular nondisplaced fractures in the elderly may also require only cast immobilization, although the patient is advised that some residual arthritis may occur.[16] For other displaced fractures or intra-articular radial fractures in young patients, treatments such as percutaneous pinning or open reduction internal fixation may be required to minimize long-term problems in the joint.

Carpal Fractures

Sixty percent of carpal bone fractures involve the scaphoid (or carpal navicular) bone. The injury mechanism is a fall on an outstretched hand, usually in an adolescent or young adult. The location of the fracture determines the likelihood of complications. Distal (5%) and middle (waist) scaphoid fractures (80%) carry a good prognosis for healing, whereas proximal (15%) fractures have an incidence of nonunion or avascular necrosis as high as 30% to 50% due to a poor blood supply.

Although a scaphoid fracture is usually identified on a posteroanterior view with the wrist in ulnar deviation, occasionally the fracture is not evident on the initial films. Patients with a "wrist sprain" who have tenderness over the scaphoid tubercle (palmar hand surface) or pain in the anatomic snuffbox, located between the extensor pollicis brevis and extensor pollicis longus tendons, should be immobilized in a short arm cast or splint for seven to ten days, at which time repeat films usually demonstrate the fracture. If tenderness continues but plain films remain negative, a bone scan or tomograms may be needed to confirm a suspected fracture. Because of the high risk of nonunion, scaphoid fractures require prolonged immobilization. Clinical opinion varies regarding use of a long arm cast versus a short arm cast, but in general a short arm cast applied for 8 to 12 weeks is acceptable for uncomplicated nondisplaced middle or distal fractures of the scaphoid.[16] The longer time frame is necessary to allow adequate bone healing and to prevent nonunion or avascular necrosis. For patients with a proximal fracture or for those with a treatment delay, orthopedic consultation may be wise because of the high incidence of long-term sequelae.[21] Any scaphoid fracture with displacement more than 1 mm or angulation more than 20 degrees is regarded as unstable and should also be referred for surgical treatment.

Other fractures of the carpal bones are uncommon and frequently require special radiographic views or tomograms for identification. A meticulous examination of the painful area indicates which carpal bones are likely to be involved. Because serious sequelae are common, including ulnar or median neuropathy and chronic wrist stability, orthopedic intervention is usually needed.

Wrist Instability

Although fractures of the carpal bones are unusual, sprains and other minor traumatic wrist injuries are common. A number of serious wrist injuries and carpal instabilities have been described as physicians have gained greater appreciation for the complex interactions of other ligaments and multiple articulations within the carpal complex. Roentgenography may be helpful for delineating certain problems, such as lunate and perilunate dislocations and scapholunate dissociations.[10] More sophisticated procedures, such as arthrography or MRI, may be required to identify other complex problems. Because there may be difficulty distinguishing a serious wrist injury from a minor sprain, the physician should be suspicious of wrist injuries that fail to resolve within a three- to four-week period. In these circumstances an orthopedic consultation is wise to ensure that no significant injury has been overlooked.

TFCC Injuries

The triangulofibrocartilage complex (TFCC) is a small meniscus located distal to the ulna. This tissue serves to absorb impact to forces on the ulnar aspect of the wrist. Injuries can be acute, due to a sudden impact, or chronic, due to repetitive loading such as gymnastics. As with carpal instability, the physician should be suspicious of TFCC injuries when ulnar wrist pain does not respond to three to four weeks of splinting. Orthopedic consultation, frequently with MRI, may be required to identify the specific problem.[22]

De Quervain's Tenosynovitis

A stenosing tendonitis, de Quervain's tenosynovitis, occurs in the first extensor compartment of the wrist, comprising the abductor pollicis longus and extensor pollicis brevis. As these tendons cross the radial styloid, thickness and swelling may occur. The patient complains of radial wrist pain, and there is often an occupational or vocational history of repetitive hand motion, such as knitting or sewing.

The diagnosis is confirmed by the Finkelstein test, as follows. After passive adduction of the thumb into the palm, ulnar deviation of the wrist elicits a sharp pain that reproduces the patient's symptoms. Initial treatment should include a corticosteroid injection into the tendon sheath. Other treatment options include rest, anti-inflammatory medications, and a thumb spica splint. On occasion, surgical release of the tendon sheath is required for symptomatic relief.[23]

Intersection Syndrome

Inflammation can also occur at the crossover of the first and second extensor compartments of the wrist, located 4 to 8 cm proximal to the distal radius.[24] Pain and tenderness are noted in this region, and the problem occurs as an overuse syndrome from repeated wrist extension. This anatomy should be distinguished from the more distal de Quervain's tenosynovitis. Initial treatment should include a thumb spica splint and anti-inflammatory medications. Corticosteroid injection is useful for those who do not respond to splinting.[25] This is a contrast to de Quervain's tenosynovitis where injection is the preferred initial treatment.

Carpal Tunnel Syndrome

The most common compression neuropathy of the upper extremity, carpal tunnel syndrome, is discussed in Reference 35, Chapter 67.

Hand

Metacarpal Fractures

The most common hand fracture is a "boxer's fracture" caused by impaction force and resulting in a fracture of the distal neck of the fifth metacarpal. Because of the mobility of the fourth and fifth metacarpals, volar angulation of the distal fragment of less then 40 degrees is acceptable without the need for bone manipulation.[25]

Whereas angulation is acceptable, a rotation injury around the longitudinal axis of any metacarpal necessitates orthopedic referral for surgical pinning. For a boxer's fracture with mild angulation, an ulnar gutter or volar splint with the metacarpophalangeal (MCP) joint at 90 degrees is applied for three to six weeks.[25] Midshaft fractures of the fifth metacarpal may be handled in a similar manner if angulation is less than 20 degrees. Nondisplaced fractures of the second and third metacarpals can be treated with a short arm cast, but careful physical examination must be performed to ensure that there is no rotation or angulation present, as these bone problems necessitate surgical correction. The unusual fracture that involves either the articular surface of the metacarpal base or metacarpal head mandates orthopedic consultation because of the potential for later arthritic complications.[16]

Fractures of the thumb metacarpal require surgical correction if they are intra-articular, such as Bennett's fracture (with proximal dislocation of the metacarpal) or Rolando's fracture (a comminuted intra-articular fracture of the metacarpal base). These injuries are less common than the extra-articular metacarpal fracture of the thumb, which if not angulated more than 30 degrees may be treated with a short arm thumb splint cast with the thumb in a flexed position.[26]

Infections

Palmar Hand Infections

Infections of the palmar hand surface are potential disasters. Bacteria can get underneath the dermal layer and then track along the flexor tendon sheaths. In this high glucose medium, the infection can spread rapidly and damage the flexor tendons with subsequent permanent hand impairment. Pain, tenderness, or swelling of the palmar surface suggests a deep hand infection, as does a recent history of minor trauma. Evidence of a palmar space infection mandates tetanus prophylaxis and intravenous antibiotic treatment with early orthopedic consultation for possible drainage.[27] Many physicians believe that animal bites to the palmar region of the hand warrant prophylactic antibiotic treatment to prevent complications (see Reference 35, Chapter 47).

Dorsal Hand Infections

Infections of the dorsal hand may appear worse than palmar infections because of the dramatic swelling within the loose connective tissue, but the prognosis is good. Oral antibiotics and outpatient drainage are usually satisfactory. Before treatment, however, the palmar space is inspected to ensure that the dorsal infection is not originating from a deep palmar infection that has ruptured to the dorsal surface.[27] Lacerations near the MCP joints warrant special precautions, especially those of the fourth or fifth metacarpal. The usual history for this injury is an altercation in which the patient has punched another person in the teeth and sustained a human bite, which may extend into the joint space. The patient frequently denies this history on initial questioning. If unrecognized, the subsequent infection may lead to joint destruction. When this injury is suspected, a hand surgeon should be contacted to consider operative debridement. A good rule to remember is that *all* lacerations over the MCP joints are human bites until proved otherwise.

Dupuytren's Contracture

Dupuytren's contracture, with thickening of the palmar fascia, results in asymptomatic contractures of the fingers primarily of the MCP joint.[28] The problem often starts with the ring finger and progresses slowly to include other fingers. Although the etiology is unknown, there is a familial tendency with Dupuytren's contracture occurring more frequently in middle-aged men of northern European descent. Pathologically, there is inflammation and subsequent contracture of the palmar aponeurosis, which may progress over years.[28] Although many treatment modalities have been attempted, surgical excision of the contracted region has been the most effective approach. Excision is reserved for those who have some functional hand impairment due to contracture formation.

Finger

Fractures

Distal Tip Fractures

Crush injuries to the tip of the finger cause pain because of the closed space swelling. Even when the fracture is comminuted, the fibrous septa provide stability during bone healing. Protective splinting of the tip for several weeks is usually satisfactory.[29] When fracture fragments are severely displaced, soft tissue interposition may prevent adequate healing unless surgical correction is performed. For any fracture associated with a nail bed injury, the nail bed or matrix must be repaired to minimize aberrant nail growth. Subungual hematomas, with or without an underlying fracture, can be decompressed with an electrocautery device or heated paper clip, creating a hole at the distal tip of the lunula. For any open fracture, such as a nail bed injury or drained subungual hematoma, antibiotic coverage with a cephalosporin is indicated to minimize the risk of osteomyelitis.

Middle and Proximal Phalangeal Fractures

All phalangeal fractures are examined carefully for evidence of angulation (by roentgenography) or rotation (by clinical examination).[26] Angulated or rotated phalangeal fractures are inherently unstable and require orthopedic intervention (Fig. 2.4). Nondisplaced extra-articular fractures of the middle or proximal phalanx can be managed by one to two weeks of immobilization followed by dynamic splinting with "buddy taping" to an adjacent finger.[16] Large intra-articular fractures involving the middle or proximal phalanx are usually unstable fractures. Small (<25%) avulsion fractures of the volar middle phalangeal base are frequent problems seen in the office that occur with a hyperextension injury (Fig. 2.5). In addition to the fracture is disruption of the distal insertion of the volar plate, a structure that prevents hyperextension of the proximal interphalangeal (PIP) joint. These injuries are managed by two to three weeks of immobilization with 20 to 30 degrees of flexion at the PIP joint, which allows maximal length of the collateral PIP joint ligaments and permits early finger rehabilitation. A buddy-taping program during activity or sports should continue for an additional four to six weeks. A gauze pad should be placed between the fingers in order to prevent skin maceration. Failure of the volar plate to heal properly may result in a swan-neck deformity at the PIP joint.

PIP Joint Dislocations

With sudden hyperextension the middle phalanx may dislocate dorsal to the proximal phalanx. This dislocation is easily reduced by gentle traction on the finger followed by flexion of the PIP joint. Because dislocation results in disruption of the distal volar plate, the PIP joint should then be immobilized for three to six weeks and managed as a volar plate injury as described above.[30] Lateral joint sprains with mild instability (<15 degrees of deviation) can also be managed with flexion splinting and subsequent buddy taping. Treatment of complete lateral dislocations and volar dislocations is more complex and controversial.

Tendon Injuries

Mallet Finger Injuries

Forced flexion of the distal interphalangeal (DIP) joint on an extended finger avulses the extensor tendon as it inserts into the distal phalanx, and the patient cannot extend the distal phalanx. Orthopedic referral

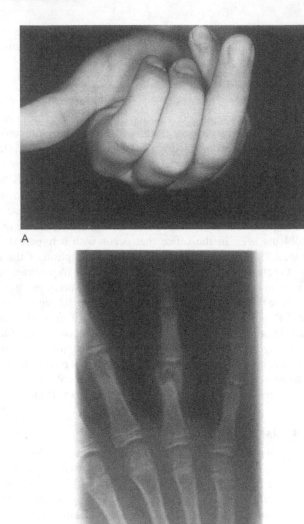

A

B

Fig. 2.4. Rotation deformity of the ring finger (A) indicates that surgical fixation is necessary to reduce the fracture. The radiograph (B), with only mild angulation, demonstrates why clinical examination for rotation is necessary for evaluating a finger injury.

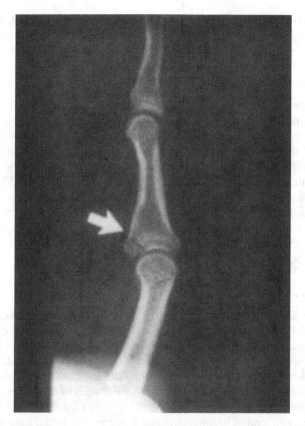

Fig. 2.5. This fracture of the middle phalanx implies that the distal volar plate has been disrupted. A combination of splinting and buddy taping for several weeks is required to allow the volar plate to heal.

is indicated only if there is subluxation of the DIP joint or if there is a large bone fragment involving more than 25% of the articular surface. Usually the roentgenogram demonstrates either no fracture or a small avulsion fragment. This injury is treated by placing the DIP joint in extension for six to eight weeks while the PIP joint is permitted to move freely.[29] A number of commercial or homemade splints are available for application to either the dorsal or volar surface of the DIP joint. Constant prolonged splinting is vital to permit tendon healing. The patient is advised that flexion of the DIP joint even once before adequate repair will result in tendon avulsion and necessitate reinitiation of the entire process. During any splint change, care is exercised to maintain finger extension. Hyperextension of the joint is also avoided, as this position may lead to necrosis of the dorsal skin.

Central Slip Injuries

A laceration or crush of the extensor tendon over the dorsum of the PIP joint or a volar dislocation damages the central portion of the extensor tendon. When this central slip is damaged, subsequent flexion of the PIP joint results in a contracture termed a boutonniere deformity. Tenderness of the central slip region is an injury of this structure until proved otherwise. A dorsal avulsion of the middle phalanx requires orthopedic pinning.[30] A potential central slip injury without fracture is treated by maintaining the PIP joint in extension for two to six weeks. The stiffness that results from collateral ligament tightening is much easier to treat than is correction of an established boutonniere deformity.

Trigger Fingers

As the flexor tendon courses through the hand, a nodular thickening at the MCP level may prevent free passage of the tendon. The cause is inflammation of the A_1 pulley, the first of five pulleys that guide the flexor tendon into the finger. Although the problem is located at the MCP level, the patient frequently complains of more distal pain at the interphalangeal (IP) joint of the thumb or PIP joint of the finger. During extension of the finger, there is a catching or locking of the PIP joint as the stenosed tendon becomes trapped in the pulley. Initial management is a tendon sheath injection with a small amount of glucocorticoid (e.g., 10 mg triamcinolone) directly into the stenosed area (Fig. 2.6). If the trigger finger persists, surgical release is necessary.[31]

Gamekeeper's Thumb

Damage to the ulnar collateral ligament that occurs with sudden hyperabduction is termed a gamekeeper's or skier's thumb. This ligament is vital for open grasp and pinch action of the hand. Swelling and tenderness of the ulnar side of the MCP joint suggest this injury. A roentgenogram of the thumb is obtained to ensure there is no fracture before the MCP joint is tested. To examine for instability, the MCP joint is stressed with the IP joint of the thumb in both extension and flexion.[16] An unstable joint or a roentgenogram that shows a large avulsion fragment necessitates orthopedic referral for possible

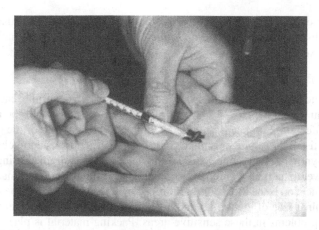

Fig. 2.6. Injection of a trigger finger is performed into the A$_1$ pulley at the MCP level. The needle can be directed proximally (as shown) or distally.

surgical exploration. Often the interposition of an adductor aponeurosis between the ends of the torn ligament (termed a Stener lesion) prevents ligament healing unless surgery is performed. Early repair of the ligament, within one to two weeks, optimizes return of hand function. If there is tenderness but the MCP joint is stable, a thumb spica splint or cast is applied for two to four weeks and the joint then reassessed for instability.

Infections

Paronychia

A nail bed infection, paronychia is often introduced by minor trauma such as manicuring or nail biting. Redness and swelling occur along the nail folds, and fluctuance is common. Treatment involves a scalpel incision between the nail fold and the nail plate with evacuation of pus; a finger block before incision is optional. The incision is made parallel to the nail plate to avoid damage to the germinal nail matrix. In the unusual event of a subungual abscess, more extensive surgery with partial nail removal is required to drain the abscess. Because an acute paronychia usually involves *Staphylococcus aureus* a short course (five to seven days) of an antistaphylococcal antibiotic is often included. Chronic paronychia is often associated with occupational water exposure, such as by dishwashers or bartenders.[32] The infecting organism is usually *Candida albicans*. Treatment usually includes nail excision.

Felon

Infection of the distal pulp space, or felon, is usually painful because of swelling within a closed space. Minor trauma often provides the nidus for infection. Surgical drainage is required to prevent loss of the entire pulp tissue or to prevent other complications such as osteomyelitis or tenosynovitis. Following a digital block, the felon is drained using one of several surgical techniques.[33] A lateral incision or longitudinal palmar incision is the most common. Incision of the radial side of the index and ulnar side of the thumb and little fingers is avoided to prevent sensory problems in these sensitive areas. Packing material is placed and changed frequently over the next several days, and oral antistaphylococcal antibiotics are administered while the infection resolves.

Tenosynovitis

Infection of a flexor tendon sheath, although an uncommon injury, requires early recognition to prevent serious complications. A position of finger flexion, swelling of the entire finger, and tenderness along the tendon sheath are common findings. The most specific physical finding is severe pain with passive extension of the finger, which leads one strongly to suspect flexor tenosynovitis. In sexually active patients disseminated gonorrhea may also present as tenosynovitis. Emergency orthopedic consultation is suggested for suspected tenosynovitis, as early debridement and aggressive care may allow salvage of the hand, whereas treatment delay of even 24 hours may result in a dramatic loss of finger or hand function.[34]

References

1. Paterson PD, Waters PM. Shoulder injuries in the childhood athlete. *Clin Sports Med.* 2000;19:681–91.
2. Simon RR, Koenigsknecht JJ. *Emergency Orthopedics: The Extremities*, 3rd ed. Norwalk, CT: Appleton & Lange, 1995;199–215.
3. Miches WF, Rodriquez RA, Amy E. Joint and soft tissue injections of the upper extremity. *Phys Med Rehab Clin North Am.* 1995;6:823–40.
4. Blake R, Hoffman J. Emergency department evaluation and treatment of the shoulder and humerus. *Emerg Med Clin North Am.* 1999;17:859–786.
5. Woodward TW, Best TM. The painful shoulder: Part I. Clinical evaluation. *Am Fam Physician.* 2000;61:3079–88.

6. Greenspan A. *Orthopedic Radiology: A Practical Approach*, 2nd ed. New York: Gower, 1992;5.1–5.47.
7. Cleeman E, Flatow EL. Shoulder dislocations in the young patient. *Orthop Clin North Am.* 2000;31:217–29.
8. Stayner LR, Cummings J. Should dislocations in patients older than 40 year of age. *Orthop Clin North Am.* 2000;31:231–9.
9. Woodward TW, Best TM. The painful shoulder Part II. Acute and chronic disorders. *Am Fam Physician.* 2000;61:3291–300.
10. Lebrun CM. Common upper extremity injuries. *Clin Fam Pract.* 1999;1:147–84.
11. Carter AM, Erickson SM. Proximal biceps tendon rupture. *Phys Sports Med.* 1999;27:95–101.
12. Klippel JH, ed. Rheumatoid arthritis. In: *Primer on the Rheumatic Diseases*, 11th ed. Atlanta: Arthritis Foundation, 1997; 155–61.
13. Harryman DT. Shoulders: Frozen and stiff. *Instr Course Lect.* 1993;42:247–57.
14. Sandor R. Adhesive capsulitis: Optimal treatment of frozen shoulder. *Phys Sports Med.* 2000;28:23–9.
15. Zuckerman JD, Mirabello SC, Newman D, Gallagher M, Cuomo F. The painful shoulder. Part II. Intrinsic disorders and impingement syndrome. *Am Fam Physician.* 1991;43:497–512.
16. Paras RD. Upper extremity fractures. *Clin Fam Pract.* 2000;2:637–59.
17. Shapiro MS, Wang JC. Elbow fractures: Treating to avoid complications. *Physician Sports Med.* 1995;23:39–50.
18. Thompson GH, Scoles PV. Nursemaid's elbow. In: Behrman RE, Kliegman RM, Jenson HB, eds. *Nelson Textbook of Pediatrics*, 16th ed. Philadelphia: WB Saunders, 2000;2092.
19. Simon RR, Koenigskneeht JJ. Soft tissue injuries, dislocations and disorders of the elbow and forearm. In: *Emergency Orthopedics: The Extremities*, 4th ed. New York: McGraw-Hill, 2001;253–64.
20. Kocher MS, Waters PM, Michali LJ. Upper extremity injuries in the pediatric athletic. *Sports Med.* 2000;30:117–35.
21. Rettig AC. Management of acute scaphoid fractures. *Hand Clinics.* 2000;16:381–95.
22. Buterbaugh GA, Brown TR, Horn PC. Ulnar-sided wrist pain in athletics. *Clin Sports Med.* 1998;17:567–83.
23. Rettig AC. Elbow, forearm and wrist injuries in the athlete. *Sports Med.* 1998;25:115–30.
24. Hanlon DP, Luellen JR. Intersection syndrome: A case report and review of the literature. *J Emerg Med.* 1999;17:969–71.
25. Petrizzi MJ, Petrizzi MG, Miller A. Making an ulnar gutter splint for a boxer's fracture. *Physician Sports Med.* 1999;27:111–2.
26. Lee S, Jupiter JB. Phalangeal and metacarpal fractures of the hand. *Hand Clin.* 2000;16:323–32.
27. Jebson PL. Deep subfascial space infections. *Hand Clin.* 1998;14:557–66.
28. Rayan GM. Clinical presentation and types of Dupuytren's disease. *Hand Clin.* 1999;15:87–96.
29. Wang QC, Johnson BA. Fingertip injuries. *Am Fam Physician.* 2001;63:1961–6.

30. Young CC, Raasch WG. Dislocations: Diagnosis and treatment. *Clin Fam Pract.* 2000;2:613–35.
31. Moore JS. Flexor tendon entrapment of the digits (trigger finger and trigger thumb). *J Occup Environ Med.* 2000;42:526–45.
32. Rockwell PG. Acute and chronic paronychia. *Am Fam Physician.* 2001;63:1113–6.
33. Jebson PJ. Infections of the fingertip. *Hand Clin.* 1998;14:547–55.
34. Bales SD, Schmidt CC. Pyogenic flexor tenosynovitis. *Hand Clin.* 1998;14:567–78.
35. Taylor RB, ed. *Family Medicine: Principles and Practice.* 6th ed. New York: Springer, 2003.

3
Disorders of the Lower Extremity

Kenneth M. Bielak
and Bradley E. Kocian

The lower extremities facilitate the maintenance of stature and balance, have intimate contact with the ground, and are responsible for movement over that ground. Thus injuries to the lower extremities are more frequent than those to the upper extremities. The bones and muscles of the lower extremity are relatively longer and stronger, and greater forces are required to disrupt the connections between them. This chapter provides basic information on the history, mechanism of injury, and testing procedures necessary to make an accurate diagnosis and formulate a specific management plan for injuries to the lower extremity. The common injuries are described in detail. Reference is made to uncommon and high-impact injuries that should not be missed. Other systemic disorders and sports-related and pediatric injuries are covered in other chapters, though there is some degree of overlap.

Hip and Pelvis

Hip Fractures

Aging is associated with reductions in muscle strength, increased inactivity, and a diminished sense of balance. Moreover, the presence of concomitant medical disorders and their treatments are increased, which are factors that contribute to the increased incidence of falls and fracture of the hip in those 65 years and older (see Reference 56, Chapter 24). Although hip fractures are a common malady of the elderly, anyone subjected to sufficient forces to the hip can be affected. The overall incidence approximates 250,000 hip fractures per year in the United States. In 1996 there were 340,000 hospital admissions for hip fractures in the United States.[1] Hip fractures are associated with more deaths, disability, and medical cost than all other osteoporotic fractures combined. Osteoporosis is the biggest risk factor for hip fracture. Table 3.1 outlines the major risk factors for osteoporotic hip fracture.

The incidence of hip fracture is directly related to the number of risk factors present. In one study women with low bone density and more than five risk factors (Table 3.1)[2] had a hip fracture incidence rate 27 times greater than that of women with fewer than three risk factors and normal bone density. Additionally, geometry (hip axis length) and architecture (Singh grade) further improve determination of hip fracture risk.[3] Simple measurements (reduced thickness of femoral shaft cortex, femoral neck cortex, reduction in an index of

Table 3.1. **Risk Factors for Osteoporotic Hip Fracture**

Age 80 years

Family history
Maternal hip fracture

Medical history
Any fracture since age 50
Poor health
Hyperthyroidism
Resting pulse >80 bpm

Current medication use
Anticonvulsants
Benzodiazepines
Caffeine (>2 cups of coffee per day)

Anthropometrics
Current weight less than that at age 25
Height at least 168 cm (5′ 6″) at age 25

Inadequate activity
On feet <4 hours per day
No walking for exercise
Inability to rise from chair without using one's arms

Visual impairment
Lowest quartile of distant depth perception (>2.44 SD)
Lowest quartile of visual contrast perception (<0.7 unit of
   contrast sensitivity)

tensile trabeculae, and wider trochanteric region) on plain radiographs were as predictive of risk for hip fracture as bone mineral density determinations.[4] Dexa scanning has become an important tool in screening for osteoporosis.

The best treatment for osteoporosis is prevention. Preventive measures include hormone replacement therapy, exercise, alendronate, increased calcium intake, and calcitonins (see Reference 56, Chapter 122). Recently, combination therapies of estrogen and alendronate have yielded even greater increases in bone mineral density and are tolerated quite well.[5] Certain facts are important to remember when considering the prescription of preventive measures: short-term intervention late in the natural course of osteoporosis may have significant effects on the incidence of hip fractures;[6] hip fracture may be associated with reduced muscle strength rather than reduced body mass or fat;[7,8] long-term heavy activity reduces the risk of hip fracture in postmenopausal women;[9] and height appears to be an important independent risk factor for hip fracture among American women and men.[10] Factors that are protective [relative risk (RR) <1] against hip fracture in the elderly are an increase in weight after age 25 and routine walking for exercise.

Fractures of the proximal femur can be classified as femoral neck, intertrochanteric, or subtrochanteric based on anatomic site. Fractures of the femoral neck (cervical or intracapsular) result from an indirect shear force on the angulated femoral neck (Fig. 3.1). They are found more commonly in the elderly and have a high risk for complications, such as avascular necrosis. Fractures of the neck of the femur are painful and can be associated with little bruising or swelling. It is important to note that a nondisplaced fracture can be ambulated upon, albeit with some degree of pain. A displaced fracture of the hip causes shortening and external rotation. Extracapsular (intertrochanteric and subtrochanteric) fractures occur with direct trauma to the hip, resulting in immediate pain, inability to ambulate, and generally significant loss of blood. In the elderly, trochanteric fractures have been associated with up to twice the short-term mortality of cervical fractures. In terms of measured bone mineral density (BMD), a relatively low trochanteric BMD or a high femoral neck BMD is associated with trochanteric hip fracture.[11] Immediate referral for orthopedic surgery is necessary. Treatment options take into account the type and extent of fracture: cervical fractures in the elderly and significant displacements require hip replacement, and extracapsular fractures respond well with repair and internal fixation.

With suspected hip fracture and negative plain radiographs, magnetic resonance imaging (MRI) demonstrated occult femoral and

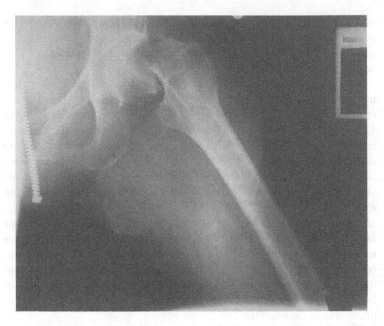

Fig. 3.1. Femoral neck fracture (intracapsular) with displacement. (Courtesy of A. Allen, M.D., Department of Radiology, University of Tennessee Medical Center.)

pelvic fractures in 37% and 23% of patients, respectively.[12] Through the use of an immediate MRI in a questionable hip fracture, the prolonged recumbency and inherent costs associated with awaiting a positive bone scan can be avoided.[13] Computed tomography (CT) scan can also be used for the diagnosis of hip fracture that is difficult to see on plain radiographs.

Hip Dislocation

Dislocation of the hip is usually the result of a motor vehicle accident or other severe trauma. Because of the relative strength of the femur in young people, hip dislocations are seen most commonly in young to middle-aged adults. Dislocations occur most commonly in the posterior direction (85–90%) but can also occur in an anterior or central direction.

The type of dislocation is largely determined by the mechanism of injury or the driving force, such as the flexed hip and knee being driven into the dashboard during a motor vehicle accident, forcing the hip to dislocate posteriorly. With a posterior hip dislocation, the physical examination shows a shortened leg that can be internally rotated and adducted. The radiographic examination includes an anteroposterior (AP) view of the pelvis (Fig. 3.2), a cross-table lateral view of the involved hip, and AP and lateral views of the involved femur to the level of the knee. An AP radiograph usually shows the femoral head superior and overlapping the acetabulum with the femur in internal rotation and adduction.[14] Complications of posterior hip dislocations include transient sciatic neuropathy, avascular necrosis, and periarticular ossification. Orthopedic referral is recommended to decrease the risk of avascular necrosis, which is directly related to the delay in reduction and the patient's age.[15] There may be associated fractures of the pelvis, femur, tibia, patella, and posterior lip of the acetabulum. Because up to 13% of radiographs do not show occult fractures, it is prudent to obtain a CT scan of the hip, if available. However, the CT scan to identify occult fractures is not necessary after reduction of simple posterior hip dislocation because it does not change the treat-

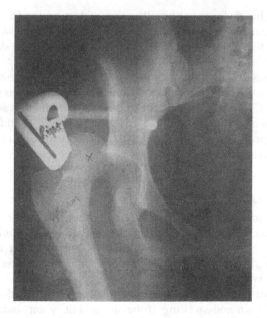

Fig. 3.2. Posterior dislocation of the right hip. Note the internal rotation and adduction of the hip with subsequent loss of the lesser trochanter silhouette. (Courtesy of A. Allen, M.D., Department of Radiology, University of Tennessee Medical Center.)

ment plan.[16] In the absence of penetrating trauma, intracapsular gas bubbles on CT are reliable indicators of recent hip dislocation and may be the only objective finding of this injury.[17] MRI can be used for the early detection of osteonecrosis of the femoral head after traumatic hip dislocation or fracture dislocation.[18]

Traumatic anterior dislocation of the hip represents 11% of all hip dislocations and is classified into superior and inferior types. Associated femoral head fractures are common, but acetabular fractures are relatively rare. Whereas inferoanterior hip dislocation is easily recognized on an anteroposterior radiograph of the pelvis, the radiographic appearance of superoanterior hip dislocation is less straightforward. Misinterpretation of a superoanterior hip dislocation can lead to an initial misdiagnosis of posterior hip dislocation, which has implications for the surgical approach and may result in failed closed reduction.[19] The superoanterior dislocation of the femoral head can be distinguished from the posterior dislocation by noting a more lateral orientation to the acetabulum and an externally rotated femur that is not adducted. The lesser trochanter becomes more prominent medially.[20]

Central hip dislocations usually occur with resulting fracture to the iliopubic portion of the acetabulum as a severe lateral blow to the hip drives the femoral head medially. There are usually other skeletal and soft tissue injuries associated with this type of injury.[14]

After closed reduction of a hip dislocation, it is necessary to confirm concentric reduction (the joint space is equidistant on plain radiograph or CT scan). The absence of concentric reduction suggests an interposition of soft tissue in the joint. Early diagnosis and treatment of this serious complication can avoid the poor results of open and deferred treatments.[21]

Pelvic Avulsion Injuries

The bony attachments of the sartorius [anterior superior iliac spine (ASIS)], rectus femoris (anterior inferior iliac spine), and the hamstrings (ischial tuberosity) can be individually avulsed by sudden overloading of the respective muscles (acute muscular contraction against a fixed resistance). The history is typically a sudden onset of extreme pain following sudden, forceful acceleration or deceleration. Localized pain and swelling at the site of injury and increased discomfort with passive stretching and muscle contraction against resistance suggest the diagnosis. Plain radiographs confirm the injury (Fig. 3.3). Subtleties may make the diagnosis obscure, and MRI may be a more sensitive and accurate way to establish the diagnosis. The ham-

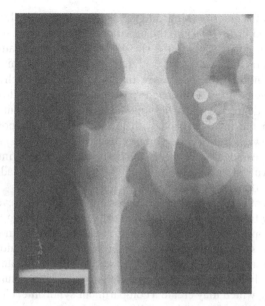

Fig. 3.3. Avulsion of the right anterior superior iliac spine (sartorius muscle origin). (Courtesy of A. Allen, M.D., Department of Radiology, University of Tennessee Medical Center.)

string avulsion may be especially common in adolescents, who have apophyses still present. Treatment of avulsion injuries is with ice, rest, and crutches with toe-touch weight-bearing for up to four to six weeks. Once the pain and swelling subside, stretching and conditioning are best provided by physical therapy before resuming regular activity to prevent formation of bony prominences at the site of injury. If there is significant displacement of the avulsed fragment, consultation with an orthopedic surgeon is recommended.

Muscle Strain, Quadriceps, Hamstring

Common mechanisms of injury to the thigh include excessive tensile forces (strain) or high-velocity compressive forces (contusions, hematoma). There can be significant overload to the quadriceps when there is forceful contraction of the knee extensor muscles against resistance. This situation commonly occurs when landing from a jump, a changing stride misstep, or catching the foot while attempting to kick a ball. The most common injury is to the rectus femoris muscle, which commonly occurs at the distal muscle–tendon unit. The rectus femoris is the most central and superficial of the quadriceps muscles of the anterior thigh, and the distal portion is the leading edge in the flexed knee. Injury to the quadriceps muscles may show a visibly swollen, tender area at the site of the muscle tear. Pain is felt on active contraction and passive stretching. Isolation of this muscle is best done in the prone position with a mild passive stretch to flexion. In the prone position, Ely's test is performed by passive flexion of the knee to 90 degrees while observing the involved hip. Spontaneous hip flexion on the involved side with this maneuver is a positive test, which shows a tight rectus femoris due to spasm or a pre-existing flexibility loss due to adaptive soft tissue changes. It is important to rule out avulsed muscles or tendons, especially to the quadriceps and patellar tendons.[22]

Treatment of muscle strain or contusion is geared to preventing further injury by decreasing the amount of bleeding by using the PRICE acronym—protection/pain-free weight bearing, rest, immobilization, ice, compressive wraps, elevation. Aspiration of the hematoma is generally not indicated, as the body resorbs this fluid, and there is increased chance for infection. If there is excessive pressure from the hematoma, which may create a compartment syndrome, elective aspiration may be performed by qualified personnel.

A quadriceps tendon rupture can occur from an off-balance jump that results in an eccentric load on a contracting muscle. Examination may reveal a large hematoma with swelling and tenderness and, possibly, a palpable defect. Incomplete tears can be managed nonoperatively with splints or hinged rehabilitation brace, crutches, and restricted weight-bearing and activity modification. Complete tears are best managed with primary surgical repair within the first 48 to 72 hours to preserve the extensor mechanism of the knee and restore function.

Contusions occur when the thigh is struck directly, resulting in muscle bruising from capillary rupture, edema, inflammation, and infiltrative bleeding. The best outcome occurs with early intervention, such as knee flexion (stretching), pain-free partial weight bearing, applying ice four to five times a day until inflammation stage is completed, restoring motion with early range of motion exercises, and subsequent aggressive rehabilitation.[23] The most troubling complication of thigh contusions is the development of myositis ossificans, which can occur in 9% to 20% of cases.[24] It can occur fairly quickly following a severe contusion with the development of tenderness, warmth, and loss of range of motion (ROM) to the involved area. If tenderness persists, radiographs obtained at three to four weeks show flocculent densities similar to a callus. Periosteal reactive changes occur in 60% of cases.[25] Calcifications leading to a mass effect with "zoning" (immature bony rim surrounding an undifferentiated highly cellular central zone)[25] are an early radiographic finding. The risk of heterotopic muscular ossification is directly related to the severity of the trauma. Milder contusions are associated with minimal risk, and severe contusions are associated with increased risk. Acute treatment is with the RICE acronym—rest, ice, compression, and elevation—with an emphasis on compression. Surgical exploration and resection of mature symptomatic heterotopic bone is usually indicated after decreased bone activity is ascertained by bone scan, usually after several months.[26]

The posterior thigh is most commonly injured by strains to the hamstrings, especially to the short head of the biceps. Hamstring strain most commonly occurs with high-velocity movements such as sprinting or hurdling maneuvers. The medial thigh is injured most commonly by strains and less so by contusions, as it is relatively more protected. The lateral thigh is most often injured by contusions because it is more exposed. An inflexible iliotibial band of the lateral thigh can be injured by strain, or chronic overuse, such as in runners on sharply curved tracks or beveled surfaces or increasing their mileage. Commonly the iliotibial band becomes inflamed by excessive friction over the lateral femoral condyle with repetitive knee flexion and extension. It is important to rule out compartment syndromes or traumatic pseudoaneurysms when dealing with injuries to the thigh.

Bursitis

The most common bursal sites that create lower extremity pain are the ischiogluteal, greater trochanter, pes anserine, medial collateral, prepatellar, popliteal, and retrocalcaneal bursae. Typically there is painful swelling that increases in intensity with prolonged weight bearing. The onset may be insidious with overuse or may be acute resulting from trauma. It is essential to rule out other more serious disorders to the underlying structures before commencing a therapeutic program.[27] Treatment consists of the PRICEMM acronym—protection, relative rest, ice, compression, elevation, medication, and modalities (e.g., ultrasonography, high-voltage electrical stimulation, or iontophoresis). Corticosteroid injections can be used effectively if one is mindful of complications such as subcutaneous fat atrophy, skin depigmentation, infection, tendon rupture, hyperglycemia, and steroid flare. It is noteworthy to remember that piriformis bursitis may cause sciatic neuropathy.

Trochanteric bursitis is typically sharply localized over the greater trochanter, and relief of pain after an injection of anesthetic and steroid confirms the diagnosis. Etiologic factors include malalignment of the lower extremity, leg length asymmetry, gluteus medius weakness, and inflexibility of the iliotibial band. Achilles tendonitis is inflammation overlying the Achilles tendon. It can be caused by rubbing the heel against an offending heel counter from new shoes, overtraining, overpronation, or chronically tight heel cords. The examiner finds tenderness, variable swelling, discomfort with movement, and possibly crepitation along the distal tendon. Treatment is to remove the cause by using a temporary $1/4$-inch heel lift, ice, nonsteroidal antiinflammatory drugs (NSAIDs), and iontophoresis or phonophoresis (ultrasonic waves to drive antiinflammatory medication toward the site of injury). Retrocalcaneal bursitis is distinctly different in that the site of inflammation is located anterior to the Achilles tendon at its insertion into the calcaneus. Typically, the shoe is the culprit due to chronic friction, and shoe modification is needed. Additional treatment is similar to that for Achilles tendonitis.

The clinical diagnosis of pes anserine bursitis is based on tenderness over the insertion of the tendons onto the medial tibia (gracilis, sartorius, semitendinosus aponeurosis) along with swelling. Questionable cases ought to have an MRI to rule out other internal derangement of the knee. MRI typically shows fluid underneath the tendons of the pes anserinus at the medial aspect of the tibia near the joint line.[28]

It is important to remember that overuse inflammatory conditions of the lower extremity that occur insidiously secondary to weight-bearing stresses will have an underlying biomechanical cause. Successful treatment evolves around identifying the structural asymmetries, adaptive soft tissue changes, and gait compensations that underlie the overuse injury.

Knee Pain

There are many causes of knee pain, as outlined in Table 3.2. It is helpful to delineate knee pain by determining whether it is anterior, posterior, medial, lateral, intra-articular, or periarticular. Radiographs are usually obtained for acute traumatic knee injuries.

Meniscal Injury
Meniscal injuries are often associated with anterior cruciate ligament (ACL) tears. If a large joint effusion precludes adequate examination, prudent management calls for re-evaluation in another week or so after

Table 3.2. **Causes of Knee Pain**

Common	Uncommon	Not to be missed
Meniscal tears	Loose body intra-articularly	Stress fracture
Collateral ligament	Tibial spine avulsion	
sprains	Epiphyseal fracture	
Contusions	Popliteal cyst	
Patellofemoral	Tibial plateau fracture	
dysfunction	Popliteus tendonitis	
Patellar dislocation/	Ganglion cyst	
subluxation	Proximal tibiofibular	
Anterior cruciate	diastasis	
ligament tear	Chondromalacia patellae	
Posterior cruciate	Neuroma	
ligament tear	Osteochondritis dissecans	
Pes anserine bursitis	of the patella	
Quadriceps and	Bipartite patella	
patellar tendonitis	Synovial plica	
Patellar bursitis	Osteochondral injury	
(pre-, infra-)	Discoid meniscus	
Synovitis	Infrapatellar fat pad	
Arthritis	syndrome (Hoffa's disease)	
Plica syndrome		
Iliotibial band		
syndrome		

a course of PRICE to decrease pain and swelling. Tenderness along the joint line combined with signs of locking, catching, inability to duck walk, pain with passive hyperextension of the knee, or positive McMurray's test is highly suggestive of meniscal damage. McMurray's test is performed with the patient in the supine position and the knee in full flexion. The tibia is internally and externally rotated while placing a mild varus and valgus stress on the knee to induce entrapment of an injured meniscus, resulting in either a snap or pain. Peripheral tears of the lateral meniscus can heal spontaneously, but other meniscal tears require the attention of an orthopedic surgeon. MRI can pick up 90% to 95% of meniscal injuries. For those with contraindications for MRI, CT arthrogram can be used.

Knee Dislocation

Complete knee dislocations are infrequent but serious injuries. Most knee dislocations are associated with posterior cruciate ligament

(PCL) and ACL rupture but may occur with neither. Knee dislocation can occur with a low-velocity direct blow to the knee or high-velocity trauma such as in a motor vehicle accident, resulting in obvious distress and deformity. Because of the inherent serious trauma to the surrounding soft tissue, including nerves and blood vessels, it is imperative to act quickly and to provide for immediate transport to a hospital facility. Arteriography in the case of knee dislocation is crucial to rule out disruption of the popliteal artery. Radiography and MRI are necessary to rule out bony fragments or concomitant fracture. Neurovascular examination of the affected limb is important and is compared to the unaffected side. Prompt orthopedic referral is recommended. Treatment options can include surgical repair or immobilization for up to six weeks.

Anterior Cruciate Ligament Tear

An ACL tear can result from an external force or intrinsically, from a sudden stop, an abrupt cut, or hyperextension when the knee suddenly "gives out" (Table 3.3). There is typically a pop that is felt or heard by the individual with subsequent inability to continue the activity. A tense, bloody effusion within hours of the injury generally occurs. In the hands of an experienced clinician, more than 90% of ACL disruptions can be diagnosed at the time of injury.[29] On examination the Lachman test (an anterior drawer at 30 degrees of flexion) can confirm the diagnosis. A delay in the examination may prevent adequate diagnosis secondary to muscle spasm and severe pain. Anteroposterior, lateral, tunnel, and patellar profile radiographs are recommended to rule out other associated bone injuries. An avulsion of the proximal tibial insertion of the capsule comprises the "lateral capsule sign," or Segond's fracture. It indicates a significant injury to the lateral collateral ligament (LCL) and capsule along with a torn ACL. Occasionally in adolescents there is an avulsion of the ACL off the intercondylar tibial eminence. The degree of joint instability is related to concurrent injury and to stretching of the secondary restraining ligaments of the knee. Some individuals can return to their usual activities within two weeks after the effusion resolves. However, further stretching of the secondary ligaments can eventually result in further instability and later to disabling arthritis.

The diagnosis of partial ACL tear on clinical grounds may in reality be a complete rupture of the ACL radiographically.[30] MRI provides unequivocal evidence that ACL tears have associated injuries to the posterolateral femur and soft tissue structures of the knee that may not have been appreciated by arthroscopy alone.[31] In older relatively

Table 3.3. **Common Causes of Knee Pain and Diagnostic Pearls**

Injury	History	Examination	Investigation
ACL tear	Audible pop, giving way with twisting, cutting or forced hyperextension	Hemarthrosis (+) Lachman's (+) Pivot shift	Confirm MRI ? Lateral capsule sign ? Tibial eminence fracture
PCL tear	Direct blow to anterior tibia; forced hyperextension	Posterior tibial sag (+) Posterior drawer	? Avulsion fracture Confirm MRI
Patellar subluxation or dislocation	Giving way with knee near extension and externally rotated; direct blow	(+) Apprehension test	? Medial patellar avulsion fracture Malalignment
Collateral ligament tear	Varus or valgus stress to knee	Hemarthrosis Medial tenderness Site tenderness Pain with/without increased laxity on stress test	? Avulsion fragment Confirm MRI
Meniscal tear	Twisting injury with catching, locking, swelling	Joint-line tenderness Mild effusion ±McMurray test	Confirm with arthrogram or MRI

ACL = anterior cruciate ligament; PCL = posterior cruciate ligament.
Source: Adapted from Rothenberg MH. Evaluation of acute knee injuries. *Postgrad Med.* 1993;93:76, with permission.

inactive individuals, nonoperative treatment is a viable option, provided patients are willing to accept a modest amount of instability and an increased risk for meniscal injury and degenerative joint disease.[32] ACL-insufficient knees in active people put them at risk for early degenerative changes. When rehabilitating an ACL tear, emphasis is placed on proper alignment of the lower extremity with a 1:1 strength ratio between quadriceps and hamstrings and on improved balance and proprioception.

Posterior Cruciate Ligament Tear

The PCL can be torn by falling on a flexed knee on a hard surface or when the knee is forced into the dashboard with sudden deceleration of an automobile. There is mild swelling and discomfort with the extremes of flexion and extension of the knee as well as pain posteriorly. The posterior drawer test and the posterior "sag" sign can establish the diagnosis of an isolated tear to the PCL. MRI is an invaluable tool in the diagnosis of PCL disruptions. PCL tears associated with other ligamentous injuries may do better with operative treatment. Isolated PCL tears do reasonably well with symptomatic rest and protection until full, pain-free ROM and equal strength are back to baseline.

Ligamentous Knee Injuries

The ligaments about the knee are the primary stabilizing structures that maintain knee joint stability. The medial collateral ligament (MCL) is the weakest and therefore the most commonly injured of the three major knee stabilizers (ACL, MCL, LCL). Injury most commonly occurs to the MCL with a valgus force on a flexed knee or a direct blow to the lateral knee. MCL tears are graded I to III based on the perceived disruption of the fibers on valgus stress examination (grade I: mild, microscopic disruption; grade II: partial tear; grade III: complete disruption) as well as the degree of tenderness and swelling. Proximal tears occur more frequently than distal tears.[33] The clinical examination is most accurate within minutes of an acutely injured knee. Treatment is conservative with PRICE and return to protected activity with functional improvement.

The mechanism of ski-related ACL injuries is a combination of load forces such that there is an external rotation-valgus force combination such as when the skier catches an inside edge in the snow. Hyperextension and violent quadriceps contraction to recover from an out-of-control sitting-back posture or to gain control after landing a jump may play a role. Isolated rupture of the popliteus is considered in any patient with an acute hemarthrosis, lateral tenderness, and a stable knee, especially after an external rotation injury.[34]

Osteochondritis Dissecans of the Knee

Osteochondritis dissecans (OCD) is a condition in which a segment of bone and the overlying cartilage are separated from underlying vascularized bone. Patients present with poorly localized, aching knee pain and swelling, exacerbated by activity and twisting motions. The physical examination typically shows an intact full ROM, possibly joint effusion, and significant quadriceps atrophy. Plain radiographs with anteroposterior, lateral, axial (sunrise or merchant), and tunnel views are helpful in the diagnosis of this condition. Figure 3.4 shows an articular defect to the medial femoral condyle that is best appreciated on the lateral view. MRI is most helpful for determining the size and viability of defects as well as the stability.[35] OCD of the lateral femoral condyle or patella is referred to an orthopedic surgeon because lateral lesions tend to more weight-bearing, leading to more degenerative changes.

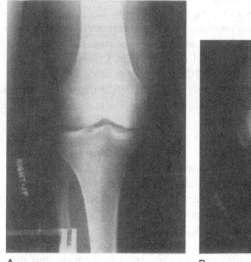
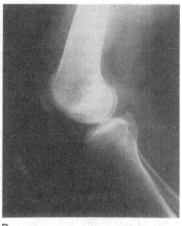

A   B

Fig. 3.4. Osteochondritis dissecans of the medial femoral condyle of right knee. Anteroposterior (A) and lateral (B) views. (Courtesy of A. Allen, M.D., Department of Radiology, University of Tennessee Medical Center.)

For most young patients brief immobilization followed by activity limitation usually results in gradual healing. "Silent" OCD lesions in the adult are treated surgically to prevent further sloughing of the bony fragment. MRI and bone scans can be reserved for patients who have not improved after four to six weeks of therapy.[35]

Osteochondral and Chondral Fractures

Osteochondral fractures are a separate entity that are often associated with ligamentous injury and penetrate the articular cartilage to the underlying subchondral bone. These fractures can result from direct trauma or a twisting injury. Patients complain of immediate pain and a snap. Osteochondral fractures can be difficult to diagnose. Multiple radiographic views are often required to isolate the injured area. Acute lesions that are nondisplaced can be treated conservatively with immobilization. Chronic lesions are best left alone unless a loose fragment is identified. It can then be removed surgically.

Chondral fractures involve injuries to the softer cartilaginous layer and are likely to be found at the lateral femoral condyle and the medial surface of the patella. Chondral fractures are found in the skeletally mature, whereas osteochondral fractures tend to be found in the skeletally immature. Diagnosis may be difficult in that the presenting history and symptoms mimic meniscal damage: a traumatic episode with the knee in flexion with subsequent effusion, locking, catching, difficulty ascending stairs, and generalized knee pain. Conservative measures of four to eight weeks of RICEMM is indicated. Those that do not resolve may need arthroscopy for a definitive diagnosis and to develop a plan for further treatment.

Patellar Dislocation

When diagnosing patellar dislocation the examiner must rule out other problems, such as ligamentous instability. Radiographic investigation is recommended (skyline and tunnel views). Patellar dislocations respond to immobilization and physical therapy. Patients with concomitant knee problems, such as predisposing patellofemoral malalignment, abnormal patellar configuration, and a history of symptoms of instability are more prone to recurrent dislocation and may benefit from operative intervention.[36] An osteochondral fragment with predisposing signs is managed operatively.[36] Up to 50% of patellar dislocations have an associated osteochondral fracture. Rehabilitation initially includes physical therapy, bracing, taping, and alteration of activities, followed by a maintenance patellar stability program.

Some injuries of the knee may be difficult to detect with simple radiographs alone. Tibial plateau fractures, Segond fractures (avulsion of the LCL from proximal tibial insertion), stress fractures, fibular head fractures, dislocation injuries to the patella and extensor mechanism, and Salter-type fractures are just a few diagnostic possibilities that may require more extensive workup with available MRI.

Lower Leg

Plantaris Tendon/Gastrocnemius Muscle Partial Tear

The tendon of the plantaris muscle can tear with violent contractions due to sudden acceleration and deceleration as is often seen on the tennis court. It is clinically difficult to differentiate between a gastrocnemius muscle tear and a plantaris tendon rupture, as they share the same anatomic location and mechanism of injury. Gastrocnemius muscle tears tend to take longer to heal. These injuries can mimic posterior compartment syndrome and deep venous thrombosis (DVT). DVT may have a palpable cord, and the compartment syndrome may have diminished distal pulses, pallor, and paresthesias. Use of Doppler ultrasonography can rule out DVT,[37] and determining intracompartment pressures can aid in ruling out compartment syndrome. Treatment consists of partial weight-bearing, if pain free, and RICE. Later, increased stretching and ROM exercises are added progressively.

Stress Fractures

Stress fractures are microscopic breaks in the cortex of long bones that have been exposed to mechanical strain due to overuse, such as with prolonged marching during military basic training. Common sites of stress fractures include the tibia, femur, and tarsal navicular and metatarsal bones.[38] Classic symptoms include persistent pain localized to a specific site that is aggravated with activity and relieved by rest and a history of recent increase in level or amount of activity. The examination may be unrevealing or may point to tenderness with compression over the site. The initial radiographs may be negative, although chronic injury may be reflected in periosteal elevation with surrounding edema. A bone scan has been historically the diagnostic procedure of choice. However, MRI has proven to be quite sensitive in diagnosing stress fractures and provides additional information such as marrow edema and actual fracture visualization. MRI is now considered the best choice for diagnosis of stress fractures for the above reasons as well as the fact that it is a noninvasive procedure.[39]

Ankle

Sprains

Ankle sprains are the most common injury to the musculoskeletal system. The lateral ankle with inversion-type mechanism of injury accounts for 85% of ankle sprains. Classification of ankle sprains is made using a grading system: grade I, mild stretch without instability; grade II, moderate stretch of the lateral ligaments resulting in partial disruption of the fibers and mild instability; and grade III, complete tear with gross instability.

Radiographic evaluation is recommended for significant injuries to rule out associated problems such as avulsion fractures, epiphyseal injuries in children, and talar dome injuries from other bony pathology that may occur. Stress radiography may be more beneficial in the chronic instability situation than in the acute setting where edema and inflammation may give a false negative. Proprioception is an important, often overlooked component during rehabilitation of an acute ankle injury and one that may have the most direct bearing on the chronic nature of ankle sprains. When treating the acute ankle sprain it is important to note that patients treated with "dynamic" bracing (protection of lateral motion while allowing full plantar and dorsiflexion) versus those with "static" bracing (i.e., immobilization and casting) have earlier, more comprehensive functional recovery.[40] Early mobilization also allows earlier return to functional capacity and may be more comfortable for the patient.[41] It takes longer to recover from syndesmosis (tibiofibular or "high ankle") sprains than from lateral ankle sprains. Complications can include ossification, which may require surgery to return to full activity.

Achilles Tendon Rupture

Seventy-five percent of Achilles tendon ruptures occur in athletes between the ages of 30 and 40 years, and two thirds are symptomatic prior to rupture. The poorest blood supply to this tendon is 2 to 6 cm proximal to its insertion, and vascularity continues to decrease with age. Risk factors include recent oral or injectable corticosteroid and chronic Achilles tendon injury. This injury usually occurs following a rapid eccentric load, with the patient feeling a "pop," as if struck from behind. There is progressive pain and inability to ambulate. Prior to swelling a palpable defect can be appreciated, and the patient cannot actively plantarflex the foot. By squeezing the relaxed prone calf, there should be movement of the foot into plantarflexion. Absence of this motion describes a positive Thomson test. A plain lateral radiograph may show either collapse of Kager's triangle (triangle formed by the borders of the anterior Achilles tendon, upper part of the calcaneus, and the posterior surface of the deep flexor tendon) or disruption of the shadow of the Achilles tendon.[42] Nonoperative treatment such as casting has recently shown similar results as operative intervention and can be considered a viable option especially in the nonelite athlete. Late ruptures are best treated surgically.[43,44]

Tibial Plafond Fractures

Fractures to the distal tibia that overlie the talus ("tenon") and comprise most of the "mortise" of the ankle joint are termed pilon fractures. The tibial plafond, or pilon fracture, occurs with 7% to 10% of tibial fractures and with only 1% of lower extremity fractures.[45] Typically pilon fractures follow a severe axial load, such as with a fall or a motor vehicle accident, but concomitant rotational forces can result in a wide array of fractures and derangements of the distal tibia and fibula. Clinically there is marked pain, swelling, inability to ambulate, and a history of severe axial loading. Because of the shear forces due to high-energy trauma associated with pilon fractures, the examiner must look for accompanying trauma to the hindfoot, knee, pelvis, and vertebral column. Nondisplaced fractures may respond favorably to casting, but most others require open reduction with internal fixation (ORIF).

Surgical reconstruction should be performed within 8 to 12 hours of injury in a stable patient without significant skin trauma; otherwise, temporizing measures to ensure restoration of length may be implemented for seven to ten days prior to ORIF.[46]

Talar Dome Fractures

Fractures to the talus account for 0.14% to 0.90% of all fractures. Because the talus contains seven articulations with adjoining structures, there is a wide variety of injury patterns to the talus: osteochondral defects to the talar dome (Fig. 3.5), posterior tubercle fractures, lateral process fractures, crush fractures, talar neck fractures, and shear fractures to the body of the talus along different planes. Often initial radiographs appear normal, but recurrent pain and instability prompt further investigation to rule out osteochondral injury to the talar dome. The symptoms of pain, recurrent swelling, ankle instability, and "giving way" are highly suggestive of osteochondritis dissecans of the talar dome (Fig. 3.5). Because bony resorption takes time to develop, follow-up radiographs may demonstrate a fracture line, sclerosis, or cyst formation. Bone scans are

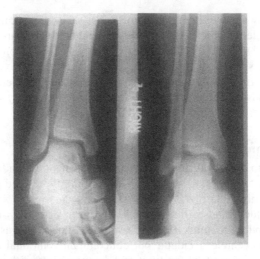

Fig. 3.5. Osteochondral injury (osteochondritis dissecans) of the lateral talar dome. (Courtesy of A. Allen, M.D., Department of Radiology, University of Tennessee Medical Center.)

undertaken if repeat radiographs are unremarkable and the history and physical examination evoke a high index of suspicion.

Staging of OCD of the talar dome is necessary for selecting the appropriate treatment option: stage I, compression of subchondral bone without break in cartilage; stage II, partially detached osteochondral fragment; stage III, totally detached osteochondral fragment remaining in crater; stage IV, displaced osteochondral fragment loose in joint.[47] Stages I, II, and III with a medial talus lesion can be managed with a short leg non-weight-bearing cast for six weeks. Referral to an orthopedic surgeon is recommended to deal with the subtleties of operative and nonoperative treatment.

Foot

Evaluation of foot injuries can be aided by classifying injuries based on the anatomic site on the hindfoot (calcaneus and talus), midfoot (tarsal bones), and forefoot (metatarsals and phalanges) (Table 3.4).

Plantar Fasciitis

Plantar fasciitis refers to disorders involving insertion of the plantar fascia into the medial tubercle of the medial calcaneus. It can present

Table 3.4. **Disorders of the Foot and Ankle**

Common	Uncommon	Not to be missed
Causes of hindfoot pain		
Plantar fasciitis	Calcaneal fracture (traumatic, stress)	Spondyloarthropathies
Fat pad contusion	Compression of the medial branch	Osteoid osteoma
	of the lateral plantar nerve	Reflex sympathetic dystrophy (RSD)
	Medial calcaneal nerve entrapment	Talar dome fracture
	Tarsal tunnel syndrome	
	Talar stress fracture	
	Retrocalcaneal bursitis	
	Haglund's deformity (pump bump)	
	Calcaneal apophysitis (Sever's disease)/(adolescents)	
	Avulsion of Achilles tendon	
	Achilles tendonitis	
Causes of midfoot pain		
Navicular stress fracture	Cuneiform stress fracture	Osteoid osteoma
Midtarsal joint sprain	Cuboid stress fracture	RSD
Extensor tendonitis	Peroneal tendonitis	
Tibialis posterior tendonitis	Abductor hallucis strain	
Plantar fascia strain	Cuboid strain	
	Tarsal coalition (adolescents)	
	Köhler's disease (young children)	

(Continued)

Table 3.4. (Continued).

Common	Uncommon	Not to be missed
Causes of forefoot pain		
Corns, calluses	Freiberg's osteochondritis	RSD
Onychocryptosis	Joplin's neuritis	Lisfranc fracture/dislocation
Synovitis MTP joints	Stress fracture sesamoids	
First MTP sprain	Toe clawing	
Subungual hematoma	Plantar wart	
Hallux valgus	Subungual exostosis	
Hallux rigidus	Hammer toe	
Morton's neuroma		
Sesamoiditis		
Metatarsal stress fracture		
Jones' fracture (5th MT base)		

MTP = metatarsophalangeal.

as an inflammation, microtear, or periosteal avulsion. Sharp heel pain is experienced with early morning ambulation and tends to lessen with activity, though a burning sensation or dull ache can occur with activity. Examination shows a specific area of tenderness overlying the medial plantar calcaneus that is aggravated by standing on the tiptoes or dorsiflexing the ankle. Tight heel cords contribute to the chronic nature of this disorder. Lateral radiographs may show heel spurs, but they are rarely the cause of the pain. Treatment options include activity modification, NSAIDs, physical therapy, heel pads, orthotic devices, night splints, and walking casts. Injectable corticosteroids are often used, but long-term efficacy is negligible. Most patients, if not all, find some lessening of symptoms during the first week. Pain relief may last as long as six to seven weeks, but more than half of these patients experience a return to preinjection discomfort.[48]

Haglund's Deformity

Haglund's deformity, or prominence of the posterosuperior os calcis, presents with pain and swelling of the heel made worse by activity. Examination by palpation reveals tenderness, thickening of the overlying skin, and signs of local inflammation. There may also be a varus deformity of the heel and a mild degree of cavus of the foot reflected by a high medial arch, making the tuberosity appear more prominent. Conservative treatment includes PRICE, and only those not benefiting from therapy are considered for surgical intervention. Surgical resection of the posterosuperior calcaneus has mixed results with little more than 50% of patients obtaining complete relief of pain.[49]

Tarsal Tunnel Syndrome

Tarsal tunnel syndrome is caused by entrapment of the posterior tibial nerve under the flexor retinaculum or at the site of either of its branches, the medial or lateral plantar nerves. The tunnel is formed by the flexor retinaculum, which is located behind and distal to the medial malleolus. Pain and paresthesias radiate along the plantar aspect of the foot from the medial malleolus and increase with activity. A positive Tinel's sign (paresthesias with percussion over the inflamed nerve) may be found along with increased discomfort from prolonged manual compression of the posterior tibial nerve behind the medial malleolus. There are many causes of this disorder, including posttraumatic deformities, tortuous veins, ganglion, lipoma, edema, the presence of accessory muscles, and synovial hypertrophy. Careful selection of candidates for resection of a space-occupying lesion has the best chance of success because of the high rate of complications and patient dissatisfaction with results.[50] MRI is helpful when planning the surgery for refractory cases of tarsal tunnel syndrome, as it identifies an inflammatory or mass lesion.[51]

Anterior Tarsal Tunnel Syndrome

Anterior tarsal tunnel syndrome is entrapment of the deep peroneal nerve (or anterior tibial nerve) under the extensor retinaculum at the ankle. The tunnel roof is the inferior extensor retinaculum; the tunnel floor is the fascia overlying the talus and navicular. Within the tunnel are four tendons, an artery, a vein, and the deep peroneal nerve. Most people with this disorder have had recurrent ankle sprains or other trauma, wear tight-fitting shoes or ski boots, carry keys under their shoelace tongue, or do sit-ups with their feet hooked under a bar. Plantar flexion with supination stretches the nerve and contributes to symptomatology. Clinical features include numbness and paresthesias in the first dorsal web space (superficial medial branch of the deep peroneal nerve) and occasionally aching and tightness about the ankle and dorsum of the foot. If the lateral, chiefly motor division of the nerve is affected, the syndrome is difficult to recognize, as the characteristic paresthesias are absent. The patient experiences only aching pain over the dorsum of the foot that is worse in some positions or less severe in others. On examination, there may be sensory loss in the first dorsal web space with a positive Tinel's sign over the area of the nerve injury, which is usually at the level of the ankle (the nerve runs a few millimeters medial to the dorsalis pedis artery). Treatment includes such conservative measures as protecting the area, rest, judicious ice, NSAIDs, and possibly surgical release of the nerve if all else fails. Table 3.5 shows other nerve impingement syndromes of the foot.[52]

Midfoot Injuries
Lisfranc Injury

The Lisfranc injury involves the articulation of the forefoot and midfoot, the tarsometatarsal joint (TMT), with or without associated fractures. This injury should be ruled out in any injury to the midfoot. The two major mechanisms of injury are direct (crushing) and the more common indirect (violent abduction or plantarflexion of the forefoot).

The midfoot sprain can be identified by mild to moderate midfoot swelling and an inability to bear weight. The TMT joint can be stressed with passive plantar and dorsiflexion, pronation, and abduction of the first and second metatarsal rays. Positive results of tenderness with these maneuvers identifies potential midfoot pathology.

Table 3.5. **Nerve Entrapment Conditions of the Foot**

Transient plantar or digital paresthetica (stair-climbing)
Classic tarsal tunnel syndrome
Distal tarsal tunnel syndromes
Medial plantar nerve
First branch of the lateral plantar nerve
Entrapment of the higher tibial nerve
Deep peroneal nerve
Superficial peroneal nerve
Sural nerve
Saphenous nerve

With no radiographic evidence of diastasis (grade III injury), treatment consists of a non-weight-bearing cast until the patient is asymptomatic. Persistent discomfort warrants a weight-bearing radiographical view to evaluate for articulation instability. The radiograph should document a space between the first and second metatarsal base that may be widened 2 to 5 mm. An ankle block may be necessary for the patient not able to tolerate weight-bearing. For more subtle injuries, diagnostic studies can be postponed for one to two weeks without a compromise in treatment. Nonoperative treatment consists of casting and the use of crutches for four to six weeks. It may take up to four months for a return to full activity.[53] Medial and global tenderness often requires a longer recovery time,[54] in contrast to injuries to the lateral aspect of the midfoot.[55] Any significant diastasis or other local soft tissue injuries require referral to an orthopedic surgeon. A history of a significant foot injury associated with persistent pain and swelling markedly out of proportion to the radiographic findings raises the suspicion of a dislocation. Comparison views with and without weight-bearing may be helpful for determining the subtle widening between the first and second metatarsal shafts.

Osteoid Osteoma

An osteoid osteoma is a benign bone lesion that can occur on any bone of the foot but is seen most often on the tarsal bones. It causes chronic pain, and one third of patients describe nocturnal pain. Many patients with osteoid osteoma fail to respond to restriction of activity. Radiography may reveal reactive cortical changes and may show a central, round, radiopaque nidus surrounded by a thin, rarefied zone usually less than 1 cm. Bone scan, CT, or MRI may add to further localization of the lesion. Referral to an orthopedic surgeon is indicated, as most of these lesions respond to local excision of the nidus.

Forefoot Injuries

Turf Toe

Hyperextension of the first metatarsophalangeal (MTP) joint or severe hallux valgus stress can result in a painful, swollen joint that becomes more severe with time. Turf toe generally refers to a sprain of the plantar capsular ligament of the big toe. Joint rest is the foremost treatment with immobilization, ice, and compression. Later, ultrasound, contrast baths, or paraffin baths offer some benefit. Taping that restricts extension of the toe may allow return to full activity.

Sesamoids

A fall from a height or forced dorsiflexion may create inflammation of the sesamoids of the foot or possibly even fracture. The pain is localized over the plantar aspect of the first metatarsal head with weight-bearing and palpation. Radiographs may show a bipartite medial sesamoid. A bone scan may be needed to rule out a stress fracture. Treatment consists of unloading the metatarsal head with padding and NSAIDs. Chronic cases may require surgery to debride or repair nonhealing fractures.

Metatarsals

The metatarsals may be injured from direct trauma, severe shear forces, and overuse. Stress fractures are common and result usually from inordinate increases in distance traveled by running or hiking. Tenderness is localized over the specific metatarsal and not within the interspace. Plain radiographs are positive within three to six weeks, but a bone scan or MRI can establish the diagnosis within days. The treatment is rest and use of a firm, flat-soled shoe. Based on symptoms, a return to activity is usually accomplished within six weeks.

Metatarsalgia

Metatarsalgia is pain under the metatarsals that is exacerbated with functional activities. It can present as burning and is more commonly seen in women and in the second metatarsal. The most common cause is increased weight-bearing pressure over the metatarsal head. It is important to rule out stress fracture, neuroma, and avascular necrosis of the metatarsal head. Treatment lies in correcting any shoe deformity that may be causing the problem; relieving the pressure point by using shoe inserts, metatarsal pads, or orthotics; and trimming any adjacent calluses. Hot soaks and NSAIDs are of proved benefit in the acute setting.

Bunion

A bunion is an excessive bony growth (exostosis) on the head of the first metatarsal with callous formation and bursal inflammation. It is the result of a tight shoe box compressing the toes or faulty foot dynamics with late pronation and push-off from the medial forefoot. Basic treatment is to find shoes with an ample toe box to decrease constriction of the MTP joint. Severe symptoms may require surgical correction. A bunionette is a bony prominence on the lateral aspect of the fifth metatarsal head.

Fracture of the Fifth Metatarsal

Fracture of the fifth metatarsal base can occur either at the base or the tuberosity. It is typically an avulsion fracture of the peroneus tendon resulting from a violent inversion stress to that side of the foot. Symptomatic treatment for three to four weeks is all that is needed prior to return to full activity. A transverse fracture at the base (Jones fracture) is associated with more complications resulting from nonunion or delayed union (Fig. 3.6). It is managed closely with immobilization. A bone graft is considered if nonunion is suspected.

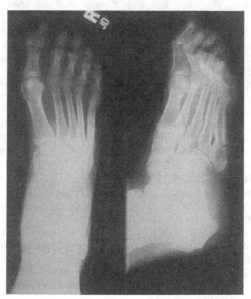

Fig. 3.6. Transverse fracture (Jones' fracture) of the base of the fifth metatarsal. (Courtesy of M. Holt, M.D., Department of Orthopedics, University of Tennessee Medical Center.)

Interdigital Neuritis (Morton's Neuroma)

Interdigital neuritis is compressive neuropathy of the interdigital nerve caused by recurrent impingement underneath the intermetatarsal ligament. It is usually seen in the third to fourth digital web space.[49] Conservative measures include rest from the offending activity, increased use of sole shock-absorbing shoes, a metatarsal pad placed proximal to the lesion, NSAIDs, or injection with anesthetic and steroids. Surgical neurolysis is used as a last resort.

References

1. Graves EJ, Owings MF. 1996 Summary: National Hospital Discharge Survey. Advance data from vital and health statistics; no. 301. Hyattsville, MD: National Center for Health Statistics, 1996.
2. Cummings SR, Browner WS, Stone K, et al. Risk factors for hip fracture in white women. *N Engl J Med*. 1995;332:767–73.
3. Peacock M, Liu G, Manatunga AK, Timmerman L, Johnston CC Jr. Better discrimination of hip fracture using bone density, geometry, and architecture. *Osteoporos Int*. 1995;5:167–73.
4. Gluer CC, Pressman A, Li J, et al. Prediction of hip fractures from pelvic radiographs: The study of osteoporotic fractures: The study of Osteoporotic Fractures Research Group. *J Bone Miner Res*. 1994; 9:671–7.
5. Lindsay R, Cosman F, Lobo RA, et al. Addition of alendronate to ongoing hormone replacement therapy in the treatment of osteoporosis: A randomized, controlled clinical trial. *J Clin Endocrinol Metab*. 1999; V84(9):3076.
6. Kanis JA, Gullberg B, Allander E, et al. Evidence for efficacy of drugs affecting bone metabolism in preventing hip fracture. *BMJ*. 1992; 305:1124–8.
7. Bean N, Lehman AB. Habitus and hip fracture revisited: Skeletal size, strength and cognition rather than thinness? *Age Ageing*. 1995;24:481–4.
8. Robinovitch SN, Hayes WC. Force attenuation in trochanteric soft tissues during impact from a fall. *J Orthop Res*. 1995;13:959–62.
9. Jaglal SB, Darlinton GA. Lifetime occupational physical activity and risk of hip fracture in women. *Ann Epidemiol*. 1995;5:321–4.
10. Hemenway D, Colditz GA. Body height and hip fracture: A cohort study of 90,000 women. *Int J Epidemiol*. 1995;24:783–6.
11. Greenspan SL, Maitland LA, Kido TH, Krasnow MB, Hayes WC. Trochanteric bone mineral density is associated with type of hip fracture in the elderly. *J Bone Miner Res*. 1994;9:1889–94.
12. Bogost GA, Cures JV III. MR imaging in evaluation of suspected hip fracture: Frequency of unsuspected bone and soft-tissue injury. *Radiology*. 1995;197:263–7.
13. Guanche CA, Kozin SH, Levy AS, Brody LA. The use of MRI in the diagnosis of occult hip fractures in the elderly: A preliminary review. *Orthopedics*. 1994;17:327–30.

14. Norris MA. Fractures and dislocations of the hip and femur. *Semin Roentgenol.* 1994;29:100–12.
15. Mitchell MJ, Resnick D. Diagnostic imaging of lower extremity trauma. *Radiol Clin North Am.* 1989;27:909–28.
16. Frick SL. Is computed tomography useful after simple posterior hip dislocation? *J Orthop Trauma.* 1995;9:388–91.
17. Fairbairn KJ, Murphey MD, Resnik CS. Gas bubbles in the hip joint on CT: an indication of recent dislocation. *AJR.* 1995;164:931–4.
18. Poggi JJ, Spritzer CE, Roark T, Goldner RD. Changes on magnetic resonance images after traumatic hip dislocation. *Clin Orthop Relat Res.* 1995;319:249–59.
19. Erb RE, Nance EP Jr, Edwards JR. Traumatic anterior dislocation of the hip: spectrum of plain film and CT findings. *AJR.* 1995;165:1215–19.
20. Rogers LF, ed. The hip and femoral shaft. In: *Radiology In Skeletal Trauma, vol. 2.* New York: Churchill Livingstone, 1992:653–712.
21. Burgos J, Ocete G. Traumatic hip dislocation with incomplete reduction due to soft-tissue interposition in a 4-year-old boy. *J Pediatr Orthop.* 1995;4:216–8.
22. Zarins B. Acute muscle and tendon injuries in athletes. *Clin Sports Med.* 1983;2:167–82.
23. Young LY, Rock MG. Thigh injuries in athletes. *Mayo Clin Proc.* 1993;68:1099–106.
24. Ryan JB, Hopkinson WJ, Arciero RA, Kolakowski KR. Quadriceps contusions. *Am J Sports Med.* 1991;19:299–304.
25. Lipscomb AB, Johnston RK. Treatment of myositis ossificans traumatica in athletes. *Am J Sports Med.* 1976;4:111–20.
26. Arrington ED. Skeletal muscle injuries. *Orthop Clin North Am.* 1995;26:411–22.
27. Butcher JD, Lillegard WA. Lower extremity bursitis. *Am Fam Physician.* 1996;53:2317–24.
28. Forbes JR, Janzen DL. Acute pes anserine bursitis: MR imaging. *Radiology.* 1995;104:525–7.
29. Johnson DL. Diagnosis for anterior cruciate ligament surgery. *Clin Sport Med.* 1993;12:671–84.
30. Lintner DM, Moseley JB, Noble PC. Partial tears of the anterior cruciate ligament. *Am J Sports Med.* 1995;23:111–6.
31. Speer KP, Bassett FH, Feagin JA, Garrett WE. Osseous injury associated with acute tears of the anterior cruciate ligament. *Am J Sports Med.* 1992;20:382–9.
32. Buss DD, Skyhar M, Galinat B, Warren RF, Wickiewicz TL. Nonoperative treatment of acute anterior cruciate ligament injuries in a selected group of patients. *Am J Sports Med.* 1995;23:160–5.
33. Schwietzer ME, Deely DM, Hume EL. Medial collateral ligament injuries: Evaluation of multiple signs, prevalence and location of associated bone bruises, and assessment with MR imaging. *Radiology.* 1995;194:825–9.
34. Geissler WB, Caspari RB. Isolated rupture of the popliteus with posterior tibial nerve palsy. *J Bone Joint Surg.* 1992;74:811–13.
35. Ralston BM, Bach BR, Bush-Joseph CA, Knopp WD. Osteochondritis dissecans of the knee. *Physician Sport Med.* 1996;24:73–84.

36. Hawkins RJ, Anisette G. Acute patellar dislocations: The natural history. *Am J Sports Med.* 1986;14:117–20.
37. Helms CA, Garvin GJ. Plantaris muscle injury: Evaluation with MR imaging. *Radiology.* 1995;195:201–3.
38. Johnson AW, Wheeler DL. Stress fractures of the femoral shaft in athletes-more common than expected. *Am J Sports Med.* 1994;22:248–56.
39. Deutsch AL, Coel MN, Mink JH. Imaging of stress injuries to bone. Radiography, scintigraphy, and MR imaging. *Clin in Sports Med.* 1997;16(2)275–91.
40. Regis D, Magnan B, Spagnol S, Bragantini A. Dynamic orthopaedic brace in the treatment of ankle sprains. *Foot Ankle Int.* 1995;16:422–6.
41. Eiff MP, Smith AT, Smith GE. Early mobilization versus immobilization in the treatment of lateral ankle sprains. *Am J Sports Med.* 1994;22:83–8.
42. Cetti R. Roentgenographic diagnoses of ruptured Achilles tendons. *Clin Orthop.* 1993;286:215–21.
43. Soma CA. Repair of acute Achilles tendon injuries. *Orthop Clin North Am.* 1995;26:239–47.
44. Howard CB, Winston I, Bell W, et al. Late repair of calcaneal tendon with carbon fiber. *J Bone Joint Surg.* 1984;66B:206–208.
45. McFerran MA, Boulas HJ. Complications encountered in the treatment of pilon fractures. *J Orthop Trauma.* 1992;6:195–200.
46. Brumback RJ. Fractures of the tibial plafond. *Orthop Clin North Am.* 1995;26:273–85.
47. Berndt AL. Transchondral fractures (osteochondritis dissecans) of the talus. *J Bone Joint Surg.* 1959;41A:988–1020.
48. Miller RA, McGuire M. Efficacy of first time steroid injection for painful heel syndrome. *Foot Ankle Int.* 1995;16:610–2.
49. Nesse E. Poor results after resection of Haglund's heel: Analysis of 35 heels in 23 patients after 3 years. *Acta Orthop Scand.* 1994;65:107–9.
50. Pfeiffer WH. Clinical results after tarsal tunnel decompression. *J Bone Joint Surg.* 1994;76A:1222–30.
51. Frey C. Magnetic resonance imaging and the evaluation of tarsal tunnel syndrome. *Foot Ankle.* 1993;14:159–64.
52. Schon LC. Nerve entrapment, neuropathy, and nerve dysfunction in athletes. *Orthop Clin North Am.* 1994;25:47–59.
53. Shapiro MS, Finerman GAM. Rupture of Lisfranc's ligament in athletes. *Am J Sports Med.* 1994;22:687–91.
54. Trevino SG. Controversies in tarsometatarsal injuries. *Orthop Clin North Am.* 1995;26:229–38.
55. Meyer SA, Albright JP, Crowley ET, et al. Midfoot sprains in collegiate football players. *Am J Sports Med.* 1994;22:392–401.
56. Taylor RB, ed. *Family Medicine: Principles and Practice.* 6th ed. New York: Springer, 2003.

4
Osteoarthritis

Alicia D. Monroe and John B. Murphy

Epidemiology

Arthritis affects an estimated 43 million persons in the United States.[1] Osteoarthritis (OA) is the most common rheumatic disease, and the third most common principal diagnosis recorded by family practitioners for office visits made by older patients.[2,3] Hip and knee OA are a leading cause of activity limitation, disability, and dependence among the elderly.[3,4] Population-based studies of OA demonstrate that the prevalence of radiographic OA is much higher than clinically defined or symptomatic OA, and there is a progressive increase in the prevalence of OA with advancing age.[3,5] The prevalence, pattern of joint involvement, and severity of OA has been observed to vary among populations by ethnicity and race, but some of the data are conflicting. [4,6] Europeans have higher prevalence rates of radiographic hip OA (7–25%), compared to Hong Kong Chinese (1%), and Caribbean and African black populations (1–4%).[4] The National Health and Nutrition Examination Survey (NHANES I) study, showed higher rates of knee OA for U.S. black women, but no racial differences in hip OA. In the Johnson County Arthritis Study, African Americans and whites showed similar high rates of radiographic hip OA (29.9% versus 26.4%) and knee OA (37 4% versus 39.1%).[7]

Pathophysiology

Systemic factors (age, sex, race, genetics, bone density, estrogen replacement therapy, and nutritional factors) may predispose joints to local biomechanical factors (obesity, muscle weakness, joint deformity, injury) and the subsequent development of OA.[4,6] The degenerative changes seen in osteoarthritic cartilage are clearly distinct from those seen with normal aging.[8] The pathological changes in OA cartilage appear to be mediated by complex interactions between mechanical and biological factors including excessive enzymatic degradation, decreased synthesis of cartilage matrix, increased levels of cytokines and other inflammatory molecules, and dysregulation of OA chondrocytes. The net result includes disorganization of the cartilage matrix and fibrillation.[8,9] As the disease advances, disorganization gives way to fissures, erosion, ulceration, and eventually cartilage is irreversibly destroyed. As the cartilage degenerates, joint stresses are increasingly transmitted to the underlying bone, initiating the bony remodeling process, which results in marginal osteophytes, subchondral sclerosis, and cysts.

Clinical Presentation and Diagnosis

Signs and Symptoms

Osteoarthritis, classified as primary (idiopathic) or secondary, represents a "final common pathway" for a number of conditions of diverse etiologies.[6] Primary OA is further classified as localized (e.g., hands, feet, knees, or other single sites) or generalized including three or more local areas. Secondary OA is classified as (1) posttraumatic, (2) congenital or developmental, (3) metabolic, (4) endocrine, (5) other bone and joint diseases, (6) neuropathic, and (7) miscellaneous. Commonly affected joints include the interphalangeal, knee, hip, acromioclavicular, subtalar, first metatarsophalangeal, sacroiliac, temporomandibular, and carpometacarpal joint of the thumb. Joints usually spared include the metacarpophalangeal, wrist, elbow, and shoulder. Early during the symptomatic phase, OA pain is often described as a deep, aching discomfort. It occurs with motion, particularly with weight-bearing, and is relieved by rest. As the disease progresses, pain can occur with minimal motion and at rest. OA pain is typically localized to the joint, although pain associated with hip OA is often localized to the anterior inguinal region, and the medial or lateral thigh, but it may also radiate to the buttock, anterior thigh, or knee. OA pain of the spine may be associated with radicular symptoms including pain, paresthesias, and muscle weakness. Although joint stiffness can occur, it is usually of short duration (<30 minutes).

Physical examination of an affected joint may show decreased range of motion, joint deformity, bony hypertrophy, and occasionally an intra-articular effusion. Crepitance and pain on passive and active movement and mild tenderness may be found. Inflammatory changes including warmth and redness are usually absent. During late stages there may be demonstrable joint instability. Physical findings associated with hand OA include Heberden's nodes of the distal interphalangeal joints, representing cartilaginous and bony enlargement of the dorsolateral and dorsomedial aspects. Bouchard's nodes are similar findings at the proximal interphalangeal joints. Physical findings of knee OA can also include quadriceps muscle atrophy, mediolateral joint instability, limitation of joint motion, initially with extension, and varus angulation resulting from degenerative cartilage in the medial compartment of the knee. The patient with OA of the hip often holds the hip adducted, flexed, and internally rotated, which may result in functional shortening of the leg and the characteristic limp (antalgic gait).

Radiographic Features and Laboratory Findings

During early stages of OA plain radiographs may be normal. As the disease progresses, joint space narrowing becomes evident as articular cartilage is lost. Marginal osteophyte formation is seen as a result of bone proliferation. Subchondral bony sclerosis appears radiographically as increased bone density. Subchondral bone cysts develop and vary in size from several millimeters to several centimeters, appearing as translucent areas in periarticular bone. Bony deformity, joint subluxation, and loose bodies may be seen in advanced cases. Computed tomography, magnetic resonance imaging, and ultrasonography provide powerful tools for the assessment of OA, although the diagnosis of OA rarely requires such expensive modalities. There are no specific laboratory tests for OA. Unlike with the inflammatory arthritides, with OA the erythrocyte sedimentation rate (ESR) and hemogram are normal and autoantibodies are not present. If there is joint effusion, the synovial fluid is noninflammatory, with fewer than 2000 white blood cells (WBCs), a predominance of mononuclear WBCs, and a good mucin clot. The diagnosis of OA is usually based on clinical and radiologic features, with the laboratory assessment being useful for excluding other arthritic conditions or secondary causes of OA.

Management

The goals of OA management are pain control, prevention of joint damage, maximizing function and quality of life, and minimizing therapeutic toxicity.[10] An appropriate treatment plan for OA combines oral medications, exercise, and patient education. Nonpharmacological management strategies for OA include periods of rest (one to two hours) when symptoms are at their worst, avoidance of repetitive movements or static body positions that aggravate symptoms, heat (or cold) for the control of pain, weight loss if the patient is overweight, adaptive mobility aids to diminish the mechanical load on joints, adaptive equipment to assist in activities of daily living (ADL), range of motion exercises, strengthening exercises, and endurance exercises.[11,12] Immobilization should be avoided. The use of adaptive mobility aids (e.g., canes, walkers) is an important strategy, but care must be taken to ensure that the mobility aid is the correct device, properly used, appropriately sized, and in good repair. Medial knee taping to realign the patella in patients with patellofemoral OA, and the use of wedged insoles for patients with medial compartment OA and shock-absorbing footwear may help reduce joint symptoms.[10,13]

Pharmacological approaches to the treatment of OA include acetaminophen, salicylates, nonselective nonsteroidal anti-inflammatory drugs (NSAIDs), cyclooxygenase-2 (COX-2) specific inhibitors, topical analgesics, and intra-articular steroids.[14,15] Acetaminophen is advocated for use as first-line therapy for relief of mild to moderate pain, but it should be used cautiously in patients with liver disease or chronic alcohol abuse. Salicylates and NSAIDs are commonly used as first-line medications for the relief of pain related to OA. Compliance with salicylates can be a major problem given their short duration of action and the need for frequent dosing; thus NSAIDs are preferable to salicylates. There is no justification for choosing one nonselective NSAID over another based on efficacy, but it is clear that a patient who does not respond to an NSAID from one class may well respond to an NSAID from another. The choice of a nonselective NSAID versus a COX-2 specific inhibitor should be made after assessment of risk for GI toxicity (e.g., age 65 or older, history of peptic ulcer disease, previous GI bleeding, use of oral corticosteroids or anticoagulants). For patients at increased risk for upper GI bleeding, the use of a nonselective NSAID and gastroprotective therapy or a COX-2 specific inhibitor is indicated. NSAIDs should be avoided or used with extreme caution in patients at risk for renal toxicity [e.g., intrinsic renal disease, age 65 or over, hypertension, congestive heart failure, and concomitant use of diuretics or angiotensin-converting enzyme (ACE) inhibitors].[10] COX-2 inhibitors increase the risk of heart attack and stroke.

Topical capsaicin may improve hand or knee OA symptoms when added to the usual treatment; however, its use may be limited by cost and the delayed onset of effect requiring multiple applications daily and sustained use for up to four weeks. Intra-articular steroids are generally reserved for the occasional instance when there is a single painful joint or a large effusion in a single joint, and the pain is unresponsive to other modalities. For patients who do not respond to NSAIDs or acetaminophen, tramadol can be considered, but seizures have been reported as a rare side effect. Narcotics should be avoided if at all possible, but they may be considered in patients unresponsive to or unable to tolerate other medications. Glucosamine sulfate, chondroitin sulfate, or acupuncture may be effective in reducing pain symptoms from OA, and glucosamine may prevent progression of knee OA.[10,16] Osteotomy, arthroscopy, arthrodesis, and total joint

Table 4.1. **Pharmacological Treatment of Osteoarthritis**

Drug	Dosage range/frequency	Relative cost/30days
Acetaminophen	750–1000 mg qid	$
Aspirin, enteric coated	975 mg qid	$
Extended release aspirin	800 mg qid	$
Salicylic acid	3–4 g/day 2 or 3 doses	$
Choline magnesium trisalicylate	3 g/day in 1, 2, or 3 doses	$$
Celecoxib (Celebrex)	100–200mg bid	$$$$
Diclofenac (Voltaren)	150–200 mg/day in 2 or 3 doses	$$
Diflunisal (Dolobid)	500–1000 mg/day in 2 doses	$$
Etodolac (Lodine)	300 mg bid–tid	$$
Fenoprofen (Nalfon)	300–600 mg tid–qid	$$
Flurbiprofen (Ansaid)	200–300 mg/day in 2, 3, or 4 doses	$$
Ibuprofen (Motrin)	1200–3200 mg/day in 3 or 4 doses	$
Indomethacin (Indocin)	25–50 mg tid–qid	$
Ketoprofen (Orudis)	50 mg qid or 75 mg tid	$$
Meclofenamate sodium	200–400 mg in 3 or 4 doses	$$$
Meloxicam (Mobic)	7.5–15 mg/day	$$$
Nabumetone (Relafen)	1000 mg once/day to 2000 mg/day	$$$
Naproxen (Naprosyn)	250–500 mg bid–tid	$
Naproxen sodium (Anaprox)	275–550 mg bid	$
Oxaprozin (Daypro)	600–1800 mg/day	$$
Piroxicam (Feldene)	20 mg once/day	$$
Sulindac (Clinoril)	150–200 mg bid	$
Tolmetin (Tolectin)	600–1800 mg/day in 3 or 4 doses	$$

$ = 18–35; $$ = 36–55; $$$ = 56–80; $$$$ = 81–145.

replacement are the primary surgical approaches for OA. Candidates for arthroplasty are individuals with severe pain, impaired joint function, or those who have experienced declines in functional status that do not improve with nonpharmacological and pharmacological measures.

The costs of OA can be substantial (Table 4.1). The direct costs for drug therapy (which can easily exceed $60 per month)[17] are added to lost income related to time spent on physician and physical therapy visits, disability-related work absences, and absences related to surgery. The pain and functional disability associated with OA can contribute to social isolation and depression. Potentially modifiable risk factors include obesity, mechanical stress/repetitive joint usage, and joint trauma.[4] Weight reduction, avoidance of traumatic injury, prompt treatment of injury, and work-site programs designed to minimize work-related mechanical joint stress may be effective interventions for preventing OA.

References

1. CDC. Prevalence of arthritis—United States, 1997. *MMWR*. 2001; 50(17):334–6.
2. *Facts About Family Practice*. Kansas City, MO: AAFP, 1987;30–7.
3. Lawrence RC, Helmick CG, Arnett FC, et al. Estimates of the prevalence of arthritis and selected musculoskeletal disorders in the United States. *Arthritis Rheum*. 1998;41(5):778–99.
4. Felson DT, Zhang Y. An update on the epidemiology of the knee and hip osteoarthritis with a view to prevention. *Arthritis Rheum*. 1998; 41:1343–55.
5. Croft P. Review of UK data on the rheumatic diseases: Osteoarthritis. *Br J Rheumatol*. 1990;29:391–5.
6. Felson DT, conference chair. Osteoarthritis: New insights. Part I: The disease and its risk factors. *Ann Intern Med*. 2000;133:635–46.
7. Jordan JM, Linder GF, Renner JB, Fryer JG. The impact of arthritis in rural populations. *Arthritis Care Res*. 1995;8:242–50.
8. Hamerman D. The biology of osteoarthritis. *N Engl J Med*. 1989; 320:1322–30.
9. Piperno M, Reboul P, LeGraverand MH, et al. Osteoarthritic cartilage fibrillation is associated with a decrease in chrondrocyte adhesion to fibronectin. *Osteoarthritis Cartilage*. 1998;6:393–99.
10. Felson DT, conference chair. Osteoarthritis: New insights. Part 2: Treatment approaches. *Ann Intern Med*. 2000;133:726–37.
11. Dunning RD, Materson RS. A rational program of exercise for patients with osteoarthritis. *Semin Arthritis Rheum*. 1991;21(suppl 2):33–43.
12. Kovar PA, Allegrante JP, MacKenzie CR, Petersan MGE, Gutin B, Charlson ME. Supervised fitness walking in patients with osteoarthritis of the knee: a randomized controlled trial. *Ann Intern Med*. 1992;116:529–34.

13. Brandt KD. Nonsurgical management of osteoarthritis, with an emphasis on nonpharmacologic measures. *Arch Fam Med.* 1995;4:1057–64.
14. Bradley J, Brandt K, Katz B, Kalasinski L, Ryan S. Comparison of an anti-inflammatory dose of ibuprofen, an analgesic dose of ibuprofen and acetominophen in the treatment of patients with osteoarthritis. *N Engl J Med.* 1991;325:87–91.
15. Griffin MR, Brandt KD, Liang MH, Pincus T, Ray WA. Practical management of osteoarthritis: Integration of pharmacologic and nonpharmacolic measures. *Arch Fam Med.* 1995;4:1049–55.
16. Reginster JY, Deroisy R, Rovati LC, et al. Long-term effects of glucosamine sulphate on osteoarthritis progression: A randomized, placebo-controlled clinical trial. *Lancet.* 2001;357:251–56.
17. *Med Lett.* 2000;42:57–64.

5
Rheumatoid Arthritis and Related Disorders

Joseph W. Gravel Jr., Patricia A. Sereno, and Katherine E. Miller

Joint pain is a common presenting complaint to the family physician. The importance of accurate diagnosis of chronic joint pain (>6 weeks) has been even more accentuated in recent years by earlier use of drugs other than nonsteroidal anti-inflammatory drugs (NSAIDs) for treatment of rheumatoid arthritis. Continuity in the doctor–patient relationship is also particularly important, as treatment must be continually reassessed and modified over time.

Joint Pain

Differential Diagnosis

The physician's first task for a patient presenting with complaints of chronic joint pain, stiffness, redness, warmth, or swelling (in the absence of trauma) is to precisely localize the pain. Pain in small joints (hands and feet) is usually pinpointed more easily than in large joints such as the shoulder, hip, or spine. If the pain is in fact periarticular, it may be characterized as local (e.g., bursitis, tendonitis, or carpal tunnel) or diffuse (e.g., polymyalgia rheumatica, polymyositis, fibromyalgia).

If the joint pain is truly articular, the differential diagnosis is narrowed by determining whether involvement is monarticular or oligoarticular (osteoarthritis, gout, pseudogout, septic arthritis) or polyarticular. Asymmetric polyarticular arthritides include ankylosing spondylitis, psoriatic arthritis, Reiter syndrome, and spondy-loarthropathies. Symmetric polyarticular distribution suggests rheumatoid arthritis, systemic lupus erythematosus (SLE), Sjögren syndrome, polymyositis, and scleroderma. When pain is diffuse, not relatable to specific anatomic structures, or described in vague terms, fibromyalgia or psychological factors must be considered (see Chapter 6).

Correlation of joint pain with activity or at rest can differentiate inflammatory from mechanical conditions. In addition to joint pain, it is important to inquire about other symptoms, including joint stiffness, limitation of motion, swelling, weakness, and fatigue or other systemic symptoms. Stiffness is discomfort associated with joint movement after a period of inactivity. Morning stiffness and its duration (especially if >60 minutes) suggest an inflammatory arthritis such as rheumatoid arthritis, whereas patients with degenerative joint disease may complain of joint stiffness during the day rather than upon awakening. With neurological conditions such as Parkinson's disease, this stiffness tends to be relatively constant (see Reference 37, Chapter 66). Finally, constitutional symptoms such as fatigue, malaise, weight loss, and fever are common with rheumatological diseases. The patient's functional ability can be addressed by asking: "What is hard to do now that you could do before, and how does this affect your daily life?"[1] It is also useful to take an occupational history as well as inquire about hobbies or other activities requiring repetitive joint movements.

Physical Examination

A thorough physical examination is performed on all patients who present with joint pain, including the asymptomatic joints. Joints are examined for swelling, tenderness, deformity, instability, and limitation of motion. Synovial thickening or an articular effusion must be differentiated from periarticular soft tissue swelling. Joint instability can be tested by moving adjacent bones opposite to the direction they normally move; an unstable joint's adjacent bones move more than normally. Arthritic joints often have greater passive ranges of motion (ROMs) than active ROMs. The clinician must be familiar with normal ROMs to identify arthritic joints' limitations. Grip strength can be assessed with a blood pressure (BP) cuff inflated to 20 mm Hg. The maximal grip force (in millimeters of mercury) may be recorded to identify changes over time. It is also recommended to search for signs of systemic disease by looking for liver, spleen, or lymph node enlargement, neurological abnormalities, oral or nasal ulcerations, rashes, nodules, and pericardial or pulmonary rubs.

Biological factors contribute to examination variability, such as circadian changes in joint size and grip strength, among patients with rheumatoid arthritis observed over a 24-hour interval.[2] Hence it may be prudent to record the time of the examination in the medical record. Accurately recording the physical examination is important but can be cumbersome, particularly if many joints are involved. One way to address this problem is to use skeleton diagrams or draw stick figures in the medical record to illustrate involved joints.

From the history and physical examination the family physician may arrive at a short differential diagnosis of the patient's presenting joint complaints. Laboratory tests and imaging studies help to further reduce the diagnostic possibilities, but the initial history and physical examination remain the hallmarks of the diagnostic process.

Rheumatoid Arthritis

Rheumatoid arthritis (RA) is a chronic, systemic, inflammatory disease that affects mainly synovial joints in a symmetric distribution. In most patients the disease is chronic and progressive, although recent changes in the treatment of RA may serve to improve long-term outcomes. Rheumatoid arthritis occurs in all racial and ethnic groups. It is seen more commonly in women by a 3:1 ratio, and estimates of its worldwide prevalence generally are around 1%. RA occurs in all age groups but is more common with increasing age, peaking between the fourth and sixth decades of life.

The cause of RA is unknown, but there probably is not a single etiology. There appears to be a genetic predisposition, which is then triggered by unknown stimuli. This leads to proliferation of the synovial-lining cells and subsynovial vessels, forming a "pannus." Mononuclear and polymorphonuclear leukocytes invade, followed by a further inflammatory cascade involving such factors as proteases and cytokines.

Diagnosis

The diagnosis of RA is based primarily on clinical grounds rather than on the results of any gold standard test. The 1987 American College of Rheumatology (ACR) criteria for classification of RA (Table 5.1) may be used to assist the family physician with an early clinical diagnosis of RA. The temperature over RA-involved joints is often elevated, but the joints are usually not red. A pannus (caused by proliferating synovium) can sometimes be felt, as can soft tissue swelling. Early diagnosis and subsequent aggressive treatment of RA

Table 5.1. **1987 American College of Rheumatology Revised Criteria for Classification of Rheumatoid Arthritis**

Criterion	Definition
1. Morning stiffness	Morning stiffness in and around the joints lasting at least 1 hour before maximal improvement
2. Arthritis of three or more joint areas	At least three joint areas with simultaneous soft tissue swelling or fluid (not bony overgrowth alone) observed by a physician; the 14 possible joint areas are right or left PIP, MCP, wrist, elbow, knee, ankle, and MTP joints
3. Arthritis of hand joints	At least one joint area swollen as above in a wrist, MCP, or PIP
4. Symmetric arthritis	Simultaneous involvement of the same joint areas on both sides of the body; bilateral involvement of PIP, MCP, or MTP joints is acceptable without absolute symmetry
5. Rheumatoid nodules	Subcutaneous nodules over bony prominences or extensor surfaces or juxta-articular regions, observed by a physician
6. Serum rheumatoid factor	Demonstration of abnormal amounts of serum rheumatoid factor by any method that has been positive in fewer than 5% of normal control subjects.
7. Radiological changes	Radiologic changes typical of rheumatoid arthritis on posteroanterior hand and wrist roentgenograms, which must include erosions or unequivocal bony decalcification localized to or most marked adjacent to the involved joints (osteoarthritis changes alone do not qualify)

For classification of rheumatoid arthritis, at least four of these seven criteria must be met. Criteria 1 through 4 must have been present for at least six weeks. Patients with two clinical diagnoses are not excluded.

MCP = metacarpophalangeal;   MTP = metatarsophalangeal;   PIP = proximal interphalangeal.

may reduce joint destruction and disability. Patients may also demonstrate classic late changes such as swan-neck and boutonniere deformities and ulnar deviation of the metacarpophalangeal (MCP) joints due to ligamentous laxity. The swan-neck deformity is characterized by flexion of the distal interphalangeal (DIP) and MCP joints and hyperextension of the proximal interphalangeal (PIP) joint, probably due to shortening of the interosseous muscles and tendons and shortening of the dorsal tendon sheath. The boutonniere deformity results from avulsion of the extensor hood of the PIP due to chronic inflammation, causing the PIP to pop up in flexion. The DIP stays in hyperextension. Hand flexor tenosynovitis is also common with RA. Atlantoaxial (C1-2) subluxation caused by ligamentous laxity is underrecognized and is a diagnostic consideration when RA patients complain of arm or leg weakness.

Extra-Articular Manifestations

Because RA is a systemic inflammatory disease, it is not surprising that there are multiple extra-articular manifestations that help with the diagnosis; systemic symptoms such as fatigue, malaise, anorexia, weight loss, and fever may be prominent. Serious infections and hematological malignancies such as non-Hodgkin's lymphoma are also more common in patients with RA. Renal disease is usually secondary to drug toxicities or amyloidosis. RA can cause pericardial effusions, pericarditis, myocarditis, and coronary arteritis. Pulmonary complications include pleural effusions, pulmonary fibrosis, nodular lung disease, and possibly small airways disease. RA can also cause secondary Sjögren syndrome.

Subcutaneous nodules are present in 25% of patients and tend to occur in areas subject to pressure, such as the elbows and sacrum, although nodules have been found in many other areas, including (rarely) the heart and lungs. Sometimes these nodules need to be biopsied to differentiate from other entities such as gouty tophi and xanthomas.

Clinical Presentations

About 55% to 70% of patients with RA experience an insidious onset over weeks to months, 8% to 15% have an acute onset, and 15% to 20% have an intermediate onset, with symptoms developing over days to weeks.[3] Patients usually first experience small joint involvement in the hands and feet, particularly the PIPs and MCPs. Morning stiffness lasting more than one hour in these joints is suggestive of RA. Edema and inflammatory products are absorbed by lymphatics and venules with motion. Patients often have constitutional symptoms as well. Large joints become symptomatic later in the course of the disease. Symmetry of involvement is an important diagnostic feature that helps differentiate RA from other rheumatological conditions. Muscle atrophy may develop around affected joints, causing weakness out of proportion to the pain. Finally, symptoms must present for more than six weeks to establish the diagnosis.

Other less common presentations include acute-onset RA and palindromic attacks. Acute-onset RA has the best long-term prognosis. Palindromic attacks are characterized by sudden, brief episodes of swelling of a large joint such as a knee, wrist, or ankle, thereby mimicking gout. Twenty to forty percent of patients with palindromic attacks progress to the chronic joint pain of RA.[4]

Clinical Course

The course of RA ranges from an intermittent type, marked by partial or complete remissions without need for continuous therapy (approximately 20% of patients), to either rapidly or slowly progressive disease. It is unclear whether treatment alters the final result of disabling arthritis in this progressive subset of patients, although pharmacological treatment and other factors such as lowering environmental temperatures and humidity may lessen symptoms.

Laboratory Studies

Selected laboratory studies are best undertaken only after a careful history and physical examination are done. Rheumatoid factor (RF), antinuclear antibody (ANA), and erythrocyte sedimentation rate (ESR) are normally the most helpful laboratory tests to aid in the diagnosis of RA. However, positive results are not specific to RA and may be elevated with other connective tissue diseases. Furthermore, the frequency of abnormal results in the absence of disease increases with age. Thus "arthritis panels" often confuse rather than clarify the situation.

Rheumatoid factor, an immunoglobulin M (IgM) antibody, is present in 80% to 90% of patients with RA; it is usually associated with severe, advanced disease. However, between 10% and 25% of patients with RA never have an abnormal RF. ANA titers should only be ordered in patients with systemic symptoms. ANA titers may be elevated in up to 30% of patients with RA; if abnormal, it is important to entertain the diagnoses of SLE, Sjögren syndrome, and scleroderma as well. Hemolytic complements (CH_{50}), C3, and C4 are normal or increased with early RA, whereas these levels are decreased in patients with SLE. The ESR is nonspecific and a rather insensitive marker for disease activity, although it may be helpful to differentiate exacerbations from other noninflammatory etiologies. Levels of C-reactive protein (CRP) reflect RA activity and may change more rapidly than the ESR—within 24 hours rather than days or weeks.

A complete blood count (CBC) can be helpful. Many patients with RA have a chronic, mild, normochromic normocytic anemia. Most have normal white blood cell (WBC) counts. Thrombocytosis may wax and wane along with disease activity.

Finally, synovial fluid analysis in RA shows yellowish white, turbid but sterile fluid without crystals, with more than 2000 WBC/mm^3 (but typically between 10,000 and 20,000) and with more than 75% polymorphonuclear leukocytes. Synovial fluid CH_{50} is lower than that in serum, and the synovial glucose is usually at least 30 mg/dL less than the serum glucose.

Imaging Studies

Plain radiographs are not helpful for most patients early in the course of RA, as they generally show only soft tissue swelling or osteoporosis. Radiographs are indicated only to help rule out infection or fracture, when the patient has a history of malignancy, when the physical examination fails to localize the source of pain, or when pain continues despite conservative treatment. Over time, radiographs of the hands and feet in particular may show joint space narrowing, periarticular osteoporosis, and eventually marginal bony erosions.

Rheumatoid Arthritis and Osteoarthritis

Because early rheumatoid arthritis and OA (see Chapter 4) are both common entities, the family physician must often differentiate between them. With RA a predominant early symptom is morning stiffness, whereas with OA pain increases through the day and with use. Joints are symmetrically involved in RA and are usually, in order of frequency, MCPs, wrists, and PIPs; DIPs are almost never affected. OA is often less symmetric and involves weight-bearing joints (hips, knees) and DIPs. Soft tissue swelling and warmth strongly suggest RA, as do periarticular osteopenia and marginal erosions on plain films. OA patients often have bony osteophytes on physical examination or radiography more commonly than soft tissue swelling. Laboratory findings in OA are normal, whereas RA patients often have elevated ESR, RF, CRP, CH_{50}, C3, and C4, as well as anemia, eosinophilia, and thrombocytosis.

Nonpharmacological Treatment

There are numerous ways to measure treatment success for RA, including measurement of various laboratory parameters such as RF titer, ESR, and number of bony erosions on radiographs; but ultimately the patient's perception of success matters much more. The American Rheumatism Association Medical Information System (ARAMIS) and several multipurpose arthritis centers employ "the five Ds" as dimensions for describing patient outcome: death, disability, discomfort, drug toxicity, and dollar cost. Different patients value each of these outcomes differently, which the family physician must keep in mind when proposing treatment options. Optimal management of RA utilizes community resources as well as a variety of treatment modalities.

Because RA is a chronic disease with no known cure, patients often are vulnerable to quack practitioners and charlatans. With the rising popularity of the Internet, patients have access to hundreds of unregulated Web sites, many of them commercial, which advertise thousands of (often expensive) "miracle cures." Patient education and an open relationship with the family physician help protect patients from misinformation.

Concomitant anxiety and depression are common among RA patients and are important to treat. The patient's psychological status is often more influenced by control of pain, socioeconomic factors, and the patient's support mechanisms (social and family support, sense of control, and coping skills) than by changes in disease status.[5]

Rest and Exercise

Resting affected joints during periods of exacerbation, including the use of splinting, may be helpful. At other times exercise to minimize periarticular muscle atrophy is necessary, often with the help of physical and occupational therapists. Water exercise has been found to help symptoms in some patients.

Dietary Therapy

There have been many proposed diets for RA, with only a few small studies showing positive effects with specific dietary manipulations. Clearly, excessive weight places more strain on inflamed joints, and dietary recommendations can be made to promote weight loss. Diets with supplemental fatty acids to eliminate precursors of arachidonic acid (and therefore diminish leukotrienes and prostaglandins) have been proposed to help, as have fasting and vegetarian diets,[6,7] but large studies have yet to be done.

Psychological Support

The same progression of responses observed with normal grieving (shock, anger, denial, resignation, and acceptance) is seen with chronic illnesses such as RA. Patients commonly fear becoming crippled, an issue that needs to be explicitly addressed by the family physician by providing education about the disease and available treatment options. It is important to consider the diagnosis of depression, and to treat if present. Sexuality may be affected because of pain, constitutional symptoms such as fatigue, and poor self-image secondary to deformities; the patient's partner may be reluctant to engage in sexual intimacy from fear of causing discomfort. As long as it does not prevent obtaining needed treatments, acting as "normal" as possible, rather than thinking of oneself as a "rheumatoid patient," is often psychologically healthy. Families often need help coping with patients, particularly those with severe disease. If the RA patient becomes overly dependent on family or on the physician, the development of coping mechanisms will be delayed. Group psychotherapy, structured group support, and relaxation therapy, among other psychoeducational approaches, have been shown to strengthen coping strategies and to improve compliance with treatment regimens.[8]

Some particularly useful therapeutic modalities include local support groups and patient education. One specific example is the Arthritis Self-Help Course, organized by the Arthritis Foundation, which provides information on isometric exercise, relaxation techniques, joint protection, nutrition, and techniques for coping with chronic illness. The Arthritis Foundation (800-283-7800) and the National Institute of Health's National Arthritis Clearinghouse (301-495-4484) are also good sources of information for patients.

Pharmacotherapy

Pharmacological treatment of the RA patient has undergone a transformation during the last several years. Observations that radiographically detectable irreversible joint damage progresses most rapidly during the first years of RA have led to growing enthusiasm for early treatment with disease-modifying antirheumatic drugs (DMARDs). These agents may minimize synovitis and ultimately prevent irreversible joint damage.

Initiating early treatment by recognizing early signs of synovitis may be the physician's most important task. Two problems hinder the early use of these potentially valuable drugs. First, selecting the patients who should receive DMARDs and those who would do equally well with less toxic drugs is still problematic. Second, differentiating early RA from other entities is often clinically difficult and can delay treatment until after it could potentially help the most.

Aspirin and NSAIDs

There is no one consistently superior NSAID for treatment of RA. Some patients who do not respond to or tolerate a particular NSAID may respond to or better tolerate another; treatment is empiric (Table 5.2). It is important to keep in mind that aspirin-allergic asthmatic patients may develop severe bronchospasm and anaphylactoid reactions with any NSAID.[9]

An adequate trial with an NSAID requires the patient take a maximal dose for three weeks before changing to a different NSAID. It is

Table 5.2. **Common NSAIDs Used for Rheumatoid Arthritis**

Arylcarboxylic acids
  Salicylic acids
    Acetylated
      Aspirin, extended release/enteric coated
    Nonacetylated
      Diflunisal (Dolobid)
      Salsalate (Disalcid, Mono-Gesic)
Arylalkanoic acids
  Arylacetic acids
    Diclofenac (Cataflam/Voltaren)
    Naproxen (Aleve, Naprosyn)
    Naproxen sodium (Anaprox)
  Arylpropionic acids
    Ibuprofen (Advil, Motrin, Nuprin)
    Ketoprofen (Orudis)
  Oxazolepropionic acids
    Oxaprozin (Daypro)
  Heteroarylacetic acids
    Tolmetin (Tolectin)
  Indole and indene acetic acids
    Sulindac (Clinoril)
  Pyranocarboxylic acids
    Etodolac (Lodine)
Enolic acids–oxicams
  Piroxicam (Feldene)
Nonacidic agents
  Nabumetone (Relafen)
Selective COX-2 inhibitors
  Celecoxib (Celebrex)

usually best to switch to an NSAID from a different class. All NSAIDs can cause dyspepsia and gastrointestinal (GI) toxicity, and all except nonacetylated salicylates and selective cyclooxygenase-2 (COX-2) inhibitors can interfere with platelet function and prolong bleeding times. Other common side effects include renal toxicity and central nervous system (CNS) symptoms such as drowsiness, dizziness, and confusion. Misoprostol (Cytotec), a prostaglandin analogue, can prevent gastric ulceration caused by NSAIDs, although this combination has become less common since the introduction of the selective COX-2 inhibitors.[10]

Which NSAID is best to use for RA? Fries and colleagues[11] analyzed 2747 patients with RA who were followed up for an average of 3.5 years. Consistently, the least toxic NSAIDs were coated or buffered aspirin, salsalate, and ibuprofen. The most toxic were indomethacin, tolmetin sodium, meclofenamate sodium, and ketoprofen. Drugs identified in this study as having high toxicity were no more clinically effective for RA treatment than those with lower toxicity.

Cyclooxygenase-2 Inhibitors. Traditional NSAIDs inhibit both COX-1 and -2. Although COX-2 is a primary enzyme in the synthesis of prostaglandins that cause joint inflammation and pain, COX-1 leads to production of other prostaglandins, including those that are gastric-protective. Patients using selective COX-2 inhibitors experience fewer GI complications, but have similar pain relief, when compared with those using traditional NSAIDS.[12] As such, these medications are particularly useful in patients who are intolerant of the GI effects of older NSAIDs, or who are at high risk of GI complications. These drugs, however, increase the risk of heart attack and stroke.

Glucocorticoids

Glucocorticoids are used in a variety of ways for treatment of RA. Glucocorticoid articular injections are often used for temporary suppression of RA in a joint, but generally this technique is not recommended more than three times per year. Common drugs for injection include short-acting preparations such as hydrocortisone acetate; intermediate-acting preparations such as triamcinolone acetonide (Kenalog), triamcinolone diacetate (Aristocort), and methylprednisolone acetate (Depo-Medrol); and long-acting preparations such as dexa-methasone acetate (Decadron-LA), and betamethasone sodium phosphate and acetate (Celestone Soluspan). Lidocaine is usually injected with the steroid to maximize patient comfort.

Systemic glucocorticoids, most commonly prednisone, are often used as "bridge therapy," when initiating therapy with DMARDs, to keep patients comfortable for the three to six months before the DMARD takes effect. Systemic glucocorticoids may need to be continued for longer periods in patients with mostly constitutional symptoms compared to those with predominantly joint symptoms.

Low-dose prednisone may be especially useful in elderly patients as an alternative to other second-line drugs that carry more risk. Oral prednisone is given in as low a dose as is clinically effective; side effects are minimized if the dose is kept at or below 7.5 mg/day. Prednisone is usually given in a single morning dose as there is no clear advantage to dividing doses. Low-dose alternate-day therapy minimizes hypothalamic–pituitary axis suppression and infection risk, although other long-term side effects such as osteoporosis and cataract formation are unaffected.[13] Increased osteopenia probably occurs even with low-dose therapy, but measures such as vitamin D and calcium supplementation may help avoid it.

DMARDs

Radiographically detectable irreversible joint damage progresses most rapidly during the first years of RA.[14] One challenge is to develop early prognostic indicators to identify the patients who will develop severe RA and those who will not, so as to initiate needed treatment in the former group and avoid overtreatment in the latter. Evidence is growing that until these indicators are refined, in general the earlier that DMARDs are started by the family physician, usually in cooperation with a rheumatologist, the better the outcome (Table 5.3). There are few data available involving direct comparison of various DMARDs' effects on the long-term outcome of disease, and short-term trials often fail to detect significant differences.

Clinical responses to DMARDs vary considerably, ranging from complete remission to no response. Most clinicians give a trial of four to six months before changing therapy, either by increasing the dose, adding an additional DMARD, or substituting completely with a different DMARD. A relapse in symptoms usually occurs with discontinuation of these drugs, necessitating continuation even when patients are doing well. Patients often have relapses even without medication changes, necessitating frequent modification of treatment. In addition, toxic side effects may develop at any time necessitating changes in therapy.

Two of the newest DMARDs are the tumor necrosis factor (TNF) inhibitors and the pyrimidine synthesis inhibitor leflunomide. TNF is a cytokine which causes inflammation; it is present in the synovium of RA patients. TNF inhibitors have been used with good success in patients with refractory RA. However, they are expensive (a wholesale

Table 5.3. **Commonly Used Disease-Modifying Antirheumatic Drugs**

Type/generic (trade) name	Usual dosage	Toxic effects	Recommended monitoring
Gold compounds/ gold Na thiomalate (Myochrysine) Aurothioglucose (Solganal)	IM: 10 to 50 mg weekly until there is toxicity, major clinical improvement, or cumulative dose of 1 g; if effective, interval between doses is increased	Pruritus, dermatitis (up to 1/3 of patients), stomatitis, nephrotoxicity, blood dyscrasias, "nitroid" reaction: flushing, weakness, nausea, dizziness 30 min after injection	CBC, platelet count, and U/A before each to every other dose
Antimalarial/ hydroxychloroquire (Plaquenil)	PO: 400–600 mg qd with meals, when good response obtained (usually 4–12 weeks) decrease to 200–400 mg qd	Retinopathy, dermatitis, muscle weakness, hypoactive DTRs, CNS	Ophthalmological exam every 3 months (visual acuity, slit-lamp, funduscopic, visual field test), neuromuscular exam
Methotrexate (Rheumatrex)	PO: 7.5–15.0 mg weekly	Pulmonary toxicity, ulcerative stomatitis, leukopenia, thrombocytopenia, GI distress, malaise, fatigue, chills, fever, CNS, elevated LFTs/liver disease, ? Lymphoma, infection, teratogenic	CBC with platelets, LFTs weekly for 6 weeks then monthly LFTs, U/A periodically, hCG prn

(continued)

Table 5.3. (continued).

Type/generic (trade) name	Usual dosage	Toxic effects	Recommended monitoring
Azathioprine (Imuran)	PO: 50–100 mg qd, increase at 4-week intervals by 0.5mg/kg/day up to 2.4 mg/kg/day	Leukopenia, thrombocytopenia, GI, ? neoplasia if previous treatment with alkylating agents, teratogenic	CBC with platelets weekly for 1 month, 2×/month for 2 months then monthly, hCG prn
Sulfasalazine (Azulfidine)	PO: 500 mg/day, then increase up to 3 g/day	GI, skin rash, pruritus, blood dyscrasias, oligospermia	CBC, U/A q2 weeks for 3 months, then monthly for 9 months, then every 6 months.
Pyrimidine synthesis inhibitor/leflunomide (Arava)	PO: 20 mg/d	Diarrhea, rash, hepatic toxicity, teratogenic	LFTs regularly
TNF inhibitors/ etanercept (Enbrel)	SC: 25 mg twice weekly	Injection-site reaction, auto-antibody formation, infection	Only as indicated for symptoms of infection
Infliximab (Remicade)	IV: 3–10 mg/kg at 0, 2, and 6 weeks, then every 8 weeks	Headache, infusion reaction, lupuslike syndrome, infection	

CBC = complete blood count; CNS = central nervous system; DTR = deep tendon reflex; GI = gastrointestinal; hCG = human chorionic gonadotropin; LFTs = liver function tests; TNF = tumor necrosis factor; U/A = urinalysis.

cost in 2004 of $1300–1400 per month) and have common local and systemic side effects.[9]

Leflunomide has been shown to be superior to methotrexate and sulfasalazine for symptomatic relief of rheumatoid arthritis, with serious adverse effects taking place in 0% to 2% of users.[15] It is teratogenic, and female patients who want to become pregnant after having taken the drug must take cholestyramine to bind the drug. Without the cholestyramine, the medication can be present in the body for up to two years.[9]

Surgery

When pharmacological therapy and all other modalities have been attempted, surgery sometimes provides relief of pain. Ninety percent of elderly patients with severe incapacitating rheumatoid joint disease can expect excellent pain relief and satisfactory motion following total hip or knee replacement.[16]

Experimental Treatment and Therapy of the Future

Because of the chronicity, lack of a cure, and associated disability of RA, patients are vulnerable to many unproved "alternative" therapies. There is definitely a need for better therapies, making RA an intensely active area of current research.

Borrowing an idea from oncology to suppress immune responses maximally, combination therapy with DMARDs is being actively investigated. Other experimental therapies include high-dose intravenous prednisolone, total lymphoid irradiation, interferon-γ, interleukin-1 (IL-1) inhibitors, cyclosporine, monoclonal antibody antagonists against T-cell receptors, and phenytoin. Tetracyclines have been investigated for years based on the theory that infectious agents such as *Mycoplasma* or *Chlamydia* may cause RA.[17] The antibody-absorbing column Prosorba is used with plasmapheresis, and is Food and Drug Administration (FDA) approved for moderate to severe RA in patients refractory to methotrexate. It is expensive, and long-term efficacy is unknown.

Juvenile Rheumatoid Arthritis

Juvenile rheumatoid arthritis (JRA), a heterogeneous group of diseases formerly known as Still's disease, is clinically distinct from RA in adults. The cause is unknown. Hypotheses concerning etiology include infection, hypersensitivity, an autoimmune reaction, or a combination of these factors. Fortunately, at least 75% of children with

JRA eventually have long remissions without significant residual deformity or loss of function. About 5% of patients with adult RA have symptoms beginning in childhood.

Clinical manifestations of JRA fall into three major categories: pauciarticular (40–50%), polyarticular (25–40%), and systemic (10–20%). These classifications are helpful for determining diagnosis, treatment, and prognosis in children with chronic arthritis. Consideration of other possibilities for arthritis, including mechanical or degenerative disorders, septic arthritis, reactive arthritis to extra-articular infection, connective tissue diseases, neoplastic disorders, endocrine disorders (type 1 diabetes mellitus, hyperthyroidism, hypothyroidism), and idiopathic pediatric joint pain syndromes is recommended. Diagnosis may be difficult without persistent, objective joint swelling. JRA is largely a diagnosis of exclusion.

In pauciarticular-onset disease, children have four or fewer joints involved during the first six months of symptoms. Large joints are primarily affected, often asymmetrically. Pauciarticular type I JRA affects girls 80% of the time, usually before age 4. Pauciarticular type II JRA affects boys 90% of the time, usually at age 8 or older, and many go on to develop spondyloarthropathies such as ankylosing spondylitis. There is a 10% to 30% risk of chronic iridocyclitis with this disease, and many authorities recommend frequent slit-lamp examinations to prevent scarring and loss of vision.

Polyarticular-onset JRA occurs mostly in girls, involving multiple joints including small joints. RF-positive polyarticular JRA tends to be more severe than RF-negative disease, both acutely and with long-term risk of severe arthritis.

Systemic-onset JRA is characterized by high intermittent fevers (>102°F), rash, hepatosplenomegaly, lymphadenopathy, arthralgias, and leukocytosis. Arthritis becomes chronic but the systemic symptoms generally dissipate with time.

The NSAIDs are generally used as first-line treatment for JRA as concerns about Reye's syndrome have discouraged use of salicylates, the drugs of choice in the past. As in adults, low-dose methotrexate is being used more frequently as the second-line drug of choice. Sulfasalazine has also been used with success. Gold compounds and antimalarials are probably less effective in JRA than in adult RA and are used less commonly. Long-term systemic glucocorticoids are effective for symptom relief but do not prevent joint damage and are best avoided in children if possible. Topical steroids are used for associated iridocyclitis. Physical and occupational therapy are important for protecting joint mobility; this is particularly important in JRA as children often do not complain of pain but simply stop using affected joints. The ultimate goal is to utilize these various treatments to encourage children with JRA to live active, normal lives. The family physician coordinates care with other members of the treatment team and offers necessary support to the child and family.

Systemic Lupus Erythematosus

Systemic lupus erythematosus (SLE) is a complicated rheumatological disorder with a broad range of presentations. The incidence of SLE has more than tripled in the past 30 years, from 1.5/100,000 in 1950–79 to 5.6/100,000 in 1980–92.[18] The incidence among female patients is three times that of male patients, resulting in a prevalence of 1 in 700 for women between the ages of 20 and 64 years.[19,20] The disease incidence in African-American and Hispanic women in the same age group is higher than in their Caucasian counterparts.

The pathogenesis of SLE is not completely understood. Current theories include polyclonal B-cell activation and antigen stimulation resulting in the immune response that characterizes this complex disorder. Studies have pointed to a genetic factor contributing to the development of SLE. Twin studies have revealed a concordance rate among monozygotic twins to be as high as 30% to 50%. An association with human leukocyte antigen (HLA) groups DR2, DR3, DR4, and DR5 has also been found.

Laboratory Findings

Detection of antinuclear antibodies is a highly sensitive screening test for SLE, although it is not specific for SLE. A marginally elevated antinuclear antibodies titer is found in 2% to 5% of normal individuals.[20] About 95% of SLE patients have positive antinuclear antibodies titers that are more than two times higher than the normal limit identified by any given laboratory. Other antibodies identified in SLE patients include anti-double-stranded DNA, anti-DNA-histone complex, anti-Sm (Smith antigen), and anti-Ro (Robert antigen). Antibodies to dsDNA and Sm antigen are specific for SLE and have been associated with more severe cases. Anti-Ro antibodies are associated with various dermatological manifestations of SLE. Anti-single-stranded DNA is not specific for SLE and therefore plays no role in diagnosis.

Up to 30% of SLE patients also have circulating antiphospholipid antibodies. These antibodies, known as the "lupus anticoagulant" may result in prolonged partial thromboplastin (PTT) and prothrombin (PT) times yet paradoxically result in an increased risk of thrombotic events. When counseling female patients who have circulating antiphospholipid antibodies, it is important to discuss the increased risk of spontaneous abortions. In fact, a history of recurrent spontaneous midtrimester abortions should trigger testing for antiphospholipid antibodies.

Systemic lupus erythematosus is characterized by a wide variety of presentations. The SLE classification system, revised in 1982 and updated in 1997, identifies 11 symptoms of the disease or systems affected in SLE patients. To confirm a diagnosis of SLE, patients must have at least 4 of the 11 criteria present either serially or simultaneously (Table 5.4).

Mucocutaneous Manifestations

The classic malar butterfly rash is present in only one third of patients. It usually presents abruptly after exposure to sunlight and lasts for several days or weeks. More commonly, patients have a patchy maculopapular rash on sun-exposed areas. Subacute cutaneous lupus erythematosus presents with a unique rash characterized by photosensitivity and superficial, nonindurated, nonscarring lesions.

One third to two thirds of SLE patients are markedly photosensitive, and sun exposure not only results in rash but also may induce a flare of systemic manifestations. Seventy percent of patients with photosensitivity have anti-Ro antibodies.[21]

Discoid lesions are raised plaques that may result in scarring. Other skin manifestations include alopecia, hyperpigmentation, and hives. Biopsy shows immunoglobulin deposition at the dermoepidermal junction. This finding is known as the lupus band test.[22]

Arthritis

Arthralgias are the most common complaint of SLE patients and are often present at the time of initial diagnosis. Up to 76% of patients develop arthritis associated with disease activity. It is difficult to differentiate the joint complaints of SLE patients from those of RA patients, but SLE patients usually present with pain out of proportion to the degree of synovitis. Also, in contrast to RA patients, SLE patients have soft tissue involvement that can result in joint deformity without evidence of cartilage involvement (Jaccoud arthropathy). Tendon rupture can also occur.

Serositis

SLE patients can have inflammation of the pleural, pericardial, and peritoneal membranes. Exudative pleural effusions are common but

Table 5.4. **1982 American College of Rheumatology Revised Criteria for Classification of Systemic Lupus Erythematosus (updated 1997)**

Criterion	Definition
1. Malar rash	Fixed erythema, flat or raised, over the malar eminences, tending to spare the nasolabial folds
2. Discoid rash	Erythematous raised patches with adherent keratotic scaling and follicular plugging; atrophic scarring may occur in older lesions
3. Photosensitivity	Skin rash as a result of unusual reaction to sunlight, by patient history or physician observation
4. Oral ulcers	Oral or nasopharyngeal ulceration, usually painless, observed by physician
5. Arthritis	Nonerosive arthritis involving two or more peripheral joints, characterized by tenderness, swelling or effusion
6. Serositis	Pleuritis—convincing history of pleuritic pain or rub heard by a physician or evidence of pleural effusion
	OR
	Pericarditis—documented by electrocardiogram or rub or evidence of pericardial effusion
7. Renal disorder	Persistent proteinuria greater than 500 mg/24 hours or greater than 3+ on dipstick
	OR
	Cellular casts—may be red cell, hemoglobin, granular, tubular or mixed—on urine sediment
8. Neurological disorder	Seizures or psychosis in the absence of offending drugs or known metabolic derangements
9. Hematological disorder	Hemolytic anemia with reticulocytosis
	OR
	Leukopenia—less than 4000/mm^3 on 2 or more occasions
	OR
	Lymphopenia—less than 1500/mm^3 on 2 or more occasions
	OR
	Thrombocytopenia—less than 100,000/mm^3 in the absence of offending drugs

(continued)

Table 5.4. (continued).

Criterion	Definition
10. Immunological disorder	Anti-DNA in abnormal titer
	OR
	Anti-Smith antibody
	OR
	Positive finding of antiphospholipid antibodies based on:
	1. An abnormal serum level of IgG or IgM anticardiolipin antibodies
	2. A positive test result for lupus anticoagulant using a standard method
	3. A confirmed false-positive serologic test for syphilis known to be positive for at least 6 months
11. Positive ANA test	An abnormal titer of ANA by immunofluorescence or an equivalent assay at any point in time and in the absence of drugs known to be associated with drug-induced lupus syndrome.

For classification of SLE at least 4 of these 11 criteria must be met, either serially or simultaneously, during any interval of observation.

ANA = antinuclear antibody.

are usually small and therefore of little clinical importance.[22] Up to 29% of SLE patients have symptoms of pericarditis including pain, friction rub, and electrocardiographic changes.

Renal Disease

Renal involvement occurs in as many as 75% of patients, and the resulting glomerulonephritis is a major determinant of morbidity and mortality[23] (see Reference 37, Chapter 97). Immune complex deposition along the glomerular basement membrane results in an inflammatory response resulting in the characteristic glomerular findings. SLE patients should have an annual urinalysis to look for early evidence of proteinuria. Because of renal compensatory mechanisms, even urinalysis and measurement of serum creatinine or creatinine clearance may underestimate actual parenchymal damage. Renal biopsy obviously can document the type of lesion present in symptomatic patients, but biopsy results have not been useful for predicting disease progression. A persistently elevated serum creatinine level (>2 mg/dL) is the best predictor of future renal morbidity.[19]

Neurological Disorder

Neurological complaints among SLE patients vary from headache to seizures. Neuropsychiatric findings in SLE patients can be the result of direct injury from immune complexes and thrombotic events or of other organ dysfunction. Cognitive dysfunction has been documented in 20% to 70% of patients. Progressive decline in cognitive function leading to dementia has been reported but is rare. Laboratory studies in symptomatic patients are significant for antineuronal antibodies. Most patients have normal cerebrospinal fluid (CSF) findings, but CSF studies are important to exclude infectious causes of neurological manifestations. Immunological CSF studies (i.e., oligoclonal bands) are not specific in SLE patients. Studies comparing magnetic resonance imaging (MRI) to computed tomographic (CT) in symptomatic SLE patients have met with conflicting results. CT is more than adequate for diagnosing mass lesions or intracranial hemorrhage. MRI is more sensitive for picking up the signs of chronic vascular injury but may also identify incidental or clinically insignificant lesions.[23]

Hematological Disorder

It is not surprising that most SLE patients have anemia of chronic disease. Up to 25% of SLE patients may also have an autoimmune thrombocytopenia; and 5% of these patients have severe thrombocytopenia with a platelet count as low as 20,000 cells/mm.[3,23] Furthermore, SLE patients have higher incidences of both arterial and venous thromboembolic events. Some studies have shown up to a fiftyfold increase in risk of myocardial infarction among reproductive-aged women with SLE, compared to age-matched controls.[18] Some investigators have recommended prophylactic aspirin or other anticoagulation treatment for all SLE patients, regardless of antiphospholipid status,[24] and aggressive anticoagulation with warfarin [with a goal international normalized ratio (INR) of 2.5–3.5] for patients with known antiphospholipid antibodies.[18]

Treatment

Treatment of SLE is best tailored to individual patients and their specific symptoms. Current treatment regimens have in general been successful in decreasing the morbidity and mortality associated with SLE. Current data indicate that more than 90% of patients survive at least 15 years.

All SLE patients are encouraged to minimize sun exposure and to use sunscreen. The most common complaint, arthralgias, can often be adequately treated with NSAIDs. Patients being treated long term with NSAIDs should be monitored periodically for renal and hepatic side effects. Glucocorticoids have also been used to treat severe symptoms, but they increase the risk of side effects. Cutaneous manifestations of SLE generally respond well to treatment with antimalarials (i.e., hydroxychloroquine or quinacrine). For treatment of skin disease resistant to either of these agents, small studies have used dapsone, azathioprine, gold, intralesional interferon, and retinoids. Methotrexate is more effective than placebo for moderate SLE without renal involvement.[18]

The foundation of treatment of SLE patients with renal disease has long been glucocorticoid therapy; however, this practice is being challenged. Patients with mild disease can often be managed with low-dose prednisone; patients with diffuse proliferative or severe focal proliferative glomerulonephritis may require a two-month course of high-dose prednisone (1 mg/kg) followed by a prolonged taper. However, studies using cyclophosphamide have shown this drug to be effective as either a single agent or in combination with glucocorticoids, and more effective than glucocorticoids alone.[18,23]

Like treatment of renal disease, the mainstay for treating thrombocytopenia has long been glucocorticoids. Patients with disease resistant to glucocorticoid treatment may respond to splenectomy, but prior to consideration of splenectomy providers must weigh the benefits against the risks posed by decreased immune function. Cyclophosphamide and chemotherapeutic agents such as vincristine and procarbazine have also been used in patients with severe disease.[23]

Reiter Syndrome

Reiter syndrome, a form of reactive arthritis, is defined as "an acute, sterile synovitis associated with a localized infection elsewhere in the body"—generally a venereal infection.[25] The hallmark of Reiter syndrome is the triad of arthritis, conjunctivitis, and urethritis. Other symptoms found in patients with Reiter syndrome include sacroiliitis, enthesopathic symptoms with the most common sites being the Achilles' tendon and planter fascia, dactylitis, mucocutaneous lesions including stomatitis, circinate balanitis, and nail lesions.

The exact prevalence and incidence of Reiter syndrome is unknown. It has a five- to ninefold higher incidence in men and the prevalence is increased in patients positive for HLA-B27.[26] Laboratory findings in Reiter syndrome patients are usually nonspecific and do not confirm the diagnosis. There is no cure for Reiter syndrome, but the underlying illness should be treated.

Raynaud's Disease

During the late nineteenth century Maurice Raynaud described digital vasospasm that seemed to be cold-induced. He believed that this phenomenon, now known as Raynaud's disease, was due to changes in the CNS control over vascular innervation. Raynaud's phenomenon is classically described in patients who develop extremity blanching and numbness with cold exposure, followed by cyanosis and then erythema on rewarming. The fingers are affected most commonly, but the toes and ears may also be involved.

Raynaud's disease has been divided into primary and secondary forms. Primary Raynaud's is more common than the secondary form, occurring in 3% to 16% of the general population.[27] Secondary Raynaud's disease is far less common, developing in only 3% to 9% of patients; it is defined as Raynaud's phenomenon associated with the development of a connective tissue disease (most commonly scleroderma).

Evaluation of a patient in whom Raynaud's disease is suspected includes a thorough history and physical examination. Changes consistent with the disease can be reproduced in the office by immersing the patient's affected extremity in ice water. Antinuclear antibodies are positive in 17% to 26% of patients but do not predict disease progression.[28]

Investigations into the pathophysiology of Raynaud's disease have led to identification of a number of abnormalities, but the complete mechanism has not been fully established. Studies have shown that patients with this disorder have an abnormal adrenergic response. Neuropeptide release (possibly due to sensory nerve system damage) and endothelial factors have also been identified.[27–29]

It is important to discuss with patients the role of behavior modification. Conservative approaches to treatment include warm socks or mittens and cold avoidance. Patients are encouraged to stop smoking and to avoid vasoconstrictive drugs, such as amphetamines, cocaine, and over-the-counter decongestants. Caffeine may also exacerbate symptoms by causing a rebound vasoconstriction after an initial vasodilatation. In patients with vasospasm associated with emotional stress, relaxation and stress management strategies have also been helpful.

When conservative strategies fail, patients may respond to calcium channel blockers. Nifedipine has been the most widely studied at doses of 10 mg sublingually for immediate treatment of acute vasospasm or 30 to 60 mg of nifedipine taken on a chronic basis, although care must be taken to avoid symptomatic hypotension.

Scleroderma

Scleroderma, or systemic sclerosis, is a connective tissue disorder whose hallmark is tissue fibrosis. Systemic scleroderma is characterized by progressive fibrosis of the skin, lungs, heart, gastrointestinal tract, and kidneys. An association of limited skin involvement and late visceral involvement is known as CREST syndrome (*c*alcinosis, *R*aynaud's phenomenon, *e*sophageal dysmotility, *s*clerodactyly, and *t*elangiectasias). A localized form of scleroderma, known as linear scleroderma or morphea, exists when fibrotic changes are localized to the skin; it does not involve the GI tract.[30]

As with many other connective tissue diseases, scleroderma affects women three times as often as men, and the incidence in the United States is estimated to be 1/100,000 persons per year. The incidence peaks in women between the fifth and sixth decades of life.[31] Clinically, patients with systemic involvement present earlier in the disease course with mostly skin complaints.

The histopathologic features found in patients with scleroderma include diffuse small artery and arteriolar vasculitis with fibrinoid necrosis, intimal thickening, and mucopoly–saccharide deposition. The exact mechanism responsible for excess deposition is unknown.

Because there is no cure for scleroderma, treatment goals are to optimize function of involved organ systems. The skin is involved in most patients, so it is important that patients use moisturizers to help maintain skin integrity. For patients with Raynaud's phenomenon, refer to the treatment guidelines discussed above. Patients may require antihypertensive drugs and treatment for gastroesophageal reflux. Immunosuppressive agents may slow disease progression.

Sjögren Syndrome

Sjögren syndrome is a rare, chronic inflammatory autoimmune disorder characterized by the combination of keratoconjunctivitis sicca (dry eyes), xerostomia (dry mouth), and rheumatoid arthritis or connective tissue disease. Vaginal dryness is also common, and restrictive lung disease is also associated.[32] Sjögren syndrome affects women ten times more often than men. Other causes of xerostomia (i.e., drug-related) must be excluded prior to diagnosis. Unfortunately, treatment options are limited. The mainstay of treatment has long been the use of lubricants for the affected areas, as well as combined care provided by a rheumatologist, ophthalmologist, and family physician.

Ankylosing Spondylitis

Ankylosing spondylitis is an inflammatory disease of the spine that can also involve other joints and extra-articular organs. Ankylosing spondylitis is considered a seronegative spondyloarthropathy because patients with this disorder do not usually have a positive rheumatoid factor. The disease most commonly affects men (male/female ratio 5:1) and usually presents during adulthood (in the thirties). Onset after age 40 is unusual. More than 90% of Caucasian patients with ankylosing spondylitis have HLA-B27; however, it is important to remember that most patients with back pain who are positive for HLA-B27 do not have ankylosing spondylitis.

The key to diagnosis of ankylosing spondylitis is having a high clinical suspicion. More than half of the patients with ankylosing spondylitis initially present complaining of low back pain. Features that distinguish the low back pain associated with ankylosing spondylitis are morning stiffness, pain unrelieved with rest (rather, patients may try to "work the pain out"), and awakening from sleep with pain. Patients may also complain of pain in the buttocks or hips but usually do not complain of pain radiating below the knees. Many patients also have peripheral joint involvement. Large joints are more commonly involved than the small joints of the hands and feet. Enthesopathy is also common and can be demonstrated radiographically. Uveitis is a common extra-articular manifestation and often precedes joint disease.

The diagnosis can be confirmed radiographically if there is evidence of sacroiliitis. If the disease has progressed, patients have the "bamboo spine" seen on radiographs. The ESR is elevated. It is easy to measure the flexibility of the spine, which is decreased in most patients. The two most commonly used tests to assess spinal flexion are Schober's flexion test and Moll's lateral flexion test. Schober's test is performed by identifying, with the patient standing, the top of the sacrum and marking on the spine points 10 cm above this point and 5 cm below. In normal individuals, with forward flexion this distance increases by at least 5 cm. The Moll's lateral flexion test is performed by marking the point in the midaxillary line of the iliac crest and the point 20 cm above this site. When the normal patient bends to the opposite side, this distance increases by at least 3 cm.[33]

The goals of treatment of ankylosing spondylitis are to decrease pain and maintain functional status. NSAIDs are the drugs of choice to control inflammation and decrease pain. Oral prednisone has not been shown to be helpful. It is also important in the preservation of functional status to encourage the patient to strengthen back extensor muscles. At the present time, spinal ossification cannot be prevented, but function is better preserved if the patient's spine is ossified in an erect position in contrast to stooped over.

Psoriatic Arthritis

Psoriatic arthritis is a form of inflammatory arthritis seen in approximately 20% of psoriasis patients (see Reference 37, Chapter 115). Like ankylosing spondylitis, patients with psoriatic arthritis have serum negative for rheumatoid factor. Psoriatic arthritis is usually a mild form of arthritis that is sometimes difficult to distinguish from rheumatoid arthritis. Points for differentiating psoriatic arthritis from rheumatoid arthritis are as follows. Psoriatic arthritis is found in patients with psoriasis, distal joint involvement, tenosynovitis, and enthesopathy. Psoriatic arthritis is generally treated with NSAIDs or antimalarials. In up to one third of patients a flare in the skin disease may precede a flare of joint symptoms.[34]

Polymyalgia Rheumatica

Patients with polymyalgia rheumatica are usually over age 50 and present with complaints of myalgias and arthralgias referable to the hips and shoulders. The pain usually has been present for several months, and patients may suffer from constitutional symptoms including fatigue, weight loss, and low-grade fever. Patients complain that these muscles or joints are achy, and that they have morning stiffness.

Polymyalgia rheumatica has a prevalence of approximately 1 in 150 persons over age 50.[35] On clinical examination, patients are tender to palpation, but their strength is intact and creatine phosphokinase levels are normal, ruling out muscle destruction. The most characteristic finding in polymyalgia rheumatica is an elevated ESR. In fact, many patients have ESRs in excess of 100 mm/hr. It is estimated that one fourth to one half of patients with polymyalgia rheumatica also have temporal arteritis.

Some patients with polymyalgia rheumatica respond to NSAIDs, but the key to treatment has traditionally been a prolonged course of a corticosteroid. Patients generally respond quickly to prednisone at a dose of 10 to 20 mg/day. If a patient does not respond quickly to corticosteroids, consider other diagnoses. Patients often require daily steroids for a minimum of two years. When attempts are made to wean a patient off prednisone, the dose is decreased by only 1 mg/month.

Temporal Arteritis

Temporal, or giant cell, arteritis, like polymyalgia rheumatica, presents in persons over 50 years of age with an annual incidence 18/100,000 people over age 50. It is more common among the Caucasian population but has been reported in nonwhite patients; it occurs more commonly in women with a female/male ratio of 3:1. Most patients present with headache and may have tenderness to palpation over the temporal artery (see Reference 37, Chapter 63). Patients may also have visual symptoms including diplopia, hemianopia, or amaurosis fugax (visual changes usually described as a window shade being pulled down over one eye).

As with polymyalgia rheumatica, patients with temporal arteritis usually have an elevated ESR to levels higher than 100 mm/hr; confirmation of this diagnosis requires biopsy of the temporal artery. Biopsy results are more likely to be positive if specimens are obtained less than 24 hours after beginning treatment. It is recommended not to withhold treatment pending biopsy results in patients with a high clinical suspicion because of the risk of blindness. Patients are started on prednisone 1 mg/kg/day, and the dosage is decreased based on symptoms and the ESR.[36]

References

1. American College of Rheumatology Ad Hoc Committee on Clinical Guidelines. Guidelines for the initial evaluation of the adult patient with acute musculoskeletal symptoms. *Arthritis Rheum.* 1996;39:1–8.
2. Boardman PL, Hart FD. Clinical measurement of the antiinflammatory effects of salicylates in rheumatoid arthritis. *BMJ.* 1967;4:264–7.
3. Smith CA, Arnett FC. Diagnosing rheumatoid arthritis: Current criteria. *Am Fam Physician.* 1991;44:863–70.
4. Harris ED Jr. Clinical features of rheumatoid arthritis. In: Kelley WN, Harris ED Jr, Ruddy S, Sledge CB, eds. *Textbook of Rheumatology*, 5th ed. Philadelphia: Saunders, 1997;898–932.
5. Yelin E, Callahan LF. The economic cost and social and psychological impact of musculoskeletal conditions. *Arthritis Rheum.* 1995;38:1351–62.
6. Volker D, Fitzgerald P, Major G, et al. Efficacy of fish oil concentrate in the treatment of rheumatoid arthritis. *J Rheumatol.* 2000;27:2343–6.
7. Muller H, de Toledo FW, Fesch KL. Fasting followed by vegetarian diet in patients with rheumatoid arthritis: A systematic review. *Scand J Rheumatol.* 2001;30:1–10.
8. Smedstand LM, Liang, MH. Psychosocial management of rheumatic diseases. In: Kelley WN, Harris ED Jr, Ruddy S, Sledge CB, eds. *Textbook of Rheumatology*, 5th ed. Philadelphia: Saunders, 1997;534–9.
9. Abramowicz M, ed. Drugs for rheumatoid arthritis. *Med Lett.* 2000;42:57–64.
10. Graham DY, White RH, Moreland LW, et al. Duodenal and gastric ulcer prevention with misoprostol in arthritis patients taking NSAIDs. *Ann Intern Med.* 1993;119:257–61.
11. Fries JF, Williams CA, Bloch DA. The relative toxicity of nonsteroidal antiinflammatory drugs. *Arthritis Rheumatol.* 1991;34:1353–60.
12. Simon LS, Weaver AL, et al. Anti-inflammatory and upper gastrointestinal effects of celecoxib in rheumatoid arthritis: A randomized controlled trial. *JAMA.* 1999;282;1921–8.
13. Bello CS, Garrett, SD. Therapeutic and adverse effects of glucocorticoids. U.S. Pharmacist Continuing Education Program no. 430-000-99-028-H01, August 1999.
14. Van der Heijde DM, van Leeuwen MA, van Riel PL, et al. Biannual radiographic assessments of hands and feet in a three-year prospective follow-up of patients with early rheumatoid arthritis. *Arthritis Rheum.* 1992;35:26–34.
15. Shadic N. New developments in rheumatoid arthritis therapy. American College of Rheumatology anual scientific meeting, 1999.
16. Harris WH, Sledge CB. Total hip and total knee replacement. *N Engl J Med.* 1990;323:725–31,801–7.
17. Langevitz, P, Livneh A, Bank I, Pras M. Benefits of minocycline in rheumatoid arthritis. *Drug Saf.* 2000;22:405–14.
18. Ruiz-Irastorza G, Khamashta MA, Castellino G, et al. Systemic lupus erythematosus. *Lancet.* 2001;357:1027–31.
19. Mills J. Systemic lupus erythematosus. *N Engl J Med.* 1994;330:1871–9.

20. Condemi J. The autoimmune diseases. *JAMA.* 1992;268:2882–92.
21. Boumpas D, Fessier B, Austin H, et al. Systemic lupus erythematosus. Part 2. Dermatologic and joint disease, the antiphospholipid antibody syndrome, pregnancy and hormonal therapy, morbidity and mortality, and pathogenesis. *Ann Intern Med.* 1995;123:42–53.
22. Osial T, Cash J, Eisenbeis C. Arthritis associated syndromes. *Prim Care.* 1993;20:857–82.
23. Boumpas D, Austin H, Fessler B, et al. Systemic lupus erythematosus: emerging concepts. Part 1. Renal, neuropsychiatric, cardiovascular, pulmonary, and hematologic disease. *Ann Intern Med.* 1995;122:940–50.
24. Wahl DG, Bounameaux H, et al. Prophylactic antithrombotic therapy for patients with systemic lupus erythematosus with or without antiphospholipid antibodies: Do the benefits outweigh the risks? A decision analysis. *Arch Intern Med.* 2000;160(13):2042–8.
25. Hughes R, Keat A. Reiter's syndrome and reactive arthritis: A current view. *Semin Arthritis Rheum.* 1994;24(3):190–210.
26. Kirchner J. Reiter's syndrome. *Postgrad Med.* 1995;97:111–21.
27. Kahaleh B, Matucci-Cerinic M. Raynaud's phenomenon and scleroderma. *Arthritis Rheum.* 1995;38:1–4.
28. Adee A. Managing Raynaud's phenomenon: A practical approach. *Am Fam Phys.* 1993;47(4):823–9.
29. Dowd P. Raynaud's phenomenon. *Lancet.* 1995;346:283–90.
30. Sjögren R. Gastrointestinal motility disorders in scleroderma. *Arthritis Rheum.* 1994;37:1265–82.
31. Edwards J, Porter J. Raynaud's syndrome and small vessel arteriopathy. *Semin Vasc Surg.* 1993;6:56–65.
32. Lehrer S, Bogursky E, Yemmini M, et al. Gynecologic manifestations of Sjögren's syndrome. *Am J Obstet Gynecol.* 1994;170:835–7.
33. Merritt J, McLean T, Erickson R, et al. Measurement of trunk flexibility in normal subjects: Reproducibility of three clinical methods. *Mayo Clin Proc.* 1986;61:192–7.
34. Gladman D. Toward unraveling the mystery of psoriatic arthritis. *Arthritis Rheum.* 1993;36:881–3.
35. Salvarini C, Gabriel S, O'Fallon M, Hunder G. Epidemiology of polymyalgia rheumatica in Olmstead County, Minnesota, 1970–1991. *Arthritis Rheum.* 1995;38:369–73.
36. Pountain G, Hazleman B. Polymyalgia rheumatica and giant cell arteritis. *BMJ.* 1995;310:1057–9.
37. Taylor RB, ed. *Family Medicine: Principles and Practice.* 6th ed. New York: Springer, 2003.

6
Selected Disorders of the Musculoskeletal System

Jeffrey G. Jones and Doug Poplin

Problems of the Soft Tissues

Fibromyalgia

Fibromyalgia (FM) is a common musculoskeletal syndrome characterized by generalized pain, fatigue, and a number of associated symptoms. The condition has formerly been called fibrositis and psychogenic rheumatism. The condition is confusing in that there is considerable overlap between FM symptoms and those of other conditions such as myofascial pain syndrome, temporomandibular joint syndrome, and chronic fatigue syndrome.

Diagnostic Criteria

The diagnosis of FM has been standardized through the use of specific accepted diagnostic criteria (Table 6.1, Fig. 6.1).

Epidemiology

At any given time, approximately 3% to 6% of the general population meet the criteria for diagnosis of FM.[1] Studies also show that women more commonly meet the diagnostic criteria.[2] The condition most commonly begins during the thirties or forties, although it may occur at any age. There is a familial aggregation of

Table 6.1. **1990 American College of Rheumatology Diagnostic Criteria for Fibromyalgia**

1. History of widespread pain of at least 3 months' duration. This pain must be present in the axial skeleton as well as all four quadrants of the body.
2. Pain must be present in at least 11 of 18 of the following paired tender points on digital palpation.
   a. Occiput: at the suboccipital muscle insertions
   b. Cervical: at the anterior aspects of the intertransverse spaces at C5–C7
   c. Trapezius: at the midpoint of the upper border
   d. Supraspinatus: at the origins above the scapular spine near the medial border
   e. Second rib: at the second costochondral junctions
   f. Lateral epicondyle: 2 cm distal to the epicondyles
   g. Gluteal: in upper outer quadrants of buttocks in anterior fold of muscle
   h. Greater trochanter: posterior to trochanteric prominences
   i. Knees: at the medial fat pad proximal to the joint line

These points should be palpated with approximately 4 kg of pressure. For the tender point to be considered painful, the patient must state that it is painful and not merely tender.

Source: Wolfe F, Smythe HA, Yunus MB, et al. *The American College of Rheumatology 1990 Criteria for the Classification of Fibromyalgia.* 1990;33:160–72, with permission.

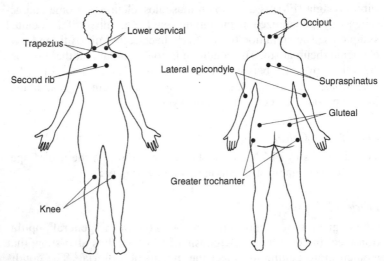

Fig. 6.1. Bilateral tender point locations in fibromyalgia are remarkably constant from patient to patient.

fibromyalgia, suggesting that there is a genetic predisposition to the condition.[3]

Clinical Features

Widespread pain and tenderness are the cardinal features of FM. Stiffness after being in one position for a prolonged period, including morning stiffness, is common. Frequently weather changes, emotional stress, unaccustomed physical activity, and menses worsen the symptoms. Although patients often report a sensation of swelling, there is usually no objective evidence of this on examination. People with FM may be more sensitive to pain throughout the body, not just in the areas of tender points. For example, it is common to see increased visceral pain in patients with FM, so associated syndromes and symptoms, such as irritable bowel syndrome, dysmenorrhea, mitral valve prolapse, interstitial cystitis, and migraine headaches are more common.[1] One must also be aware that tender points are common sites for pain even in the general population, who have an average of 3.7 positive tender points.[4] Pain perception is also influenced by a number of other factors including aerobic fitness, quality of sleep, and depression.[5] Thus a condition based on pain sensation may encompass a number of other conditions.

Most patients with FM complain of fatigue (see Reference 33, Chapter 55), and many have poor-quality sleep (see Reference 33, Chapter 56). The relation between FM and sleep disturbance is not as clear as once thought.[1] Improvement in FM symptoms with pharmacological treatment does not necessarily correlate with an improvement in sleep.[6] FM patients also have a higher incidence of migraine and tension headaches than the general population[1] (see Reference 33, Chapter 63). Approximately 84% of people with FM complain of numbness or tingling somewhere in the body.[7] Echocardiographic evidence of mitral valve prolapse is seen in up to 75% of FM patients.[8] Patients with FM have a higher incidence of depression, and controversy remains as to whether FM symptoms are a manifestation of a psychosomatic syndrome, or, conversely, depression results from chronic pain (see Reference 33, Chapters 32 and 61).

Differential Diagnosis

Early rheumatoid arthritis (and other rheumatic conditions), polymyalgia rheumatica, and hypothyroidism are included in the differential diagnosis and can generally be excluded with an appropriate history and laboratory analysis. Infections, especially human immunodeficiency virus (HIV), hepatitis, and subacute bacterial endocarditis, can also present similarly to FM. Neoplastic conditions and endocrine problems may cause similar clinical presentations.

Diagnosis

Fibromyalgia can usually be reliably diagnosed by a typical history, physical examination consistent with the appropriate number of tender points, and appropriate laboratory studies. The laboratory evaluation, which should include a thyroid-stimulating hormone (TSH) assay, erythrocyte sedimentation rate (ESR), and an antinuclear antibody (ANA) test, helps to rule out other conditions but does not rule in FM.

Management

Patient Education. Important to the management of this condition is a thorough explanation of the condition. Patients have often seen many physicians while trying to "find a cure." It is often therapeutic for patients to find a physician who can provide them with a diagnosis. The Arthritis Foundation (1314 Spring Street NW, Atlanta, GA 30309) can provide additional information.

Behavior Modification. Modifying behavior often involves emphasis on activities that help to lessen symptoms. Patients often must be reminded that caffeine, especially near bedtime, may worsen an already poor sleep pattern. Helping patients to reframe their situation into one with less victimization, along with other cognitive therapy interventions, can also be useful. Directing the patient toward self-management of symptoms through relaxation training, meditation, or electromyographic (EMG) biofeedback can help control symptoms while shifting the locus of control back to the patient.

Medication. Amitriptyline (Elavil and others) and cyclobenzaprine (Flexeril) have been studied and found to be helpful for FM. They are both tricyclic compounds, although cyclobenzaprine does not have antidepressant activities. Although it is generally acknowledged that these medicines are helpful, the mechanism of action is not clear. Low doses are recommended to start, and the doses can be slowly increased. The goal of therapy is to improve sleep and lessen symptoms but not cause a "hangover." The drugs are sometimes not well tolerated, usually due to anticholinergic side effects or vivid dreams. Zolpidem (Ambien) may be a reasonable alternative.[1] If one is not able to control symptoms with the above medicines, the selective serotonin reuptake inhibitors offer another potential option. The nonsteroidal anti-inflammatory drugs (NSAIDs) are not usually highly effective in treating this condition.

Exercise. Because it is rare for patients to have lasting improvements without exercise,[1] this modality should be emphasized in all cases.

Often these patients are deconditioned, and one must start at a low work load to avoid flaring symptoms. Water exercise classes, especially in heated pools, tend to be effective. Other exercises to consider include walking, riding stationary bicycles, and engaging in low-impact aerobics. Exercise programs that incorporate elements of muscle stretching, muscular endurance, and aerobic fitness tend to be most effective. Regardless of the specific exercise program, it must be approached slowly and consistently to produce optimal results.

Prognosis

Generally, FM patients have chronic symptoms, but their resulting disability is a function of their willingness to accept responsibility for managing these symptoms. A sense of helplessness is a strong negative predictor of outcome in FM patients.[9] Only about 5% of FM patients have a complete remission.[10] Patients may need to be guided away from costly and untested treatments. Patients should be counseled vocationally into returning to nonphysically demanding work. As with many other chronic conditions, the empathetic, optimistic physician's guidance and support can be therapeutic and help to empower FM patients to cope effectively with their conditions.

Myofascial Pain Syndrome

Definition

Myofascial pain syndrome (MPS) is the name given to the common clinical syndrome of persistent regional or local pain in muscle(s) accompanied by "trigger points" on palpation of the involved muscles. The trigger point has local tenderness, the presence of a "taut band," and a twitch response. Palpation of the trigger point characteristically produces pain referred beyond it.[11] The syndrome may be acute and is often seen after strain or trauma to a muscle. Nonmusculoskeletal symptoms, such as fatigue, are unusual. The pathophysiology is not well understood.

The terminology used to describe this and related problems is not standardized, adding to the confusion. Many authors see MPS as an entity distinct from FM, although there is some thought that MPS and FM represent two extremes of a single disorder.[12] It is not unusual for a patient to have symptoms characteristic of both syndromes.

Clinical Features

Patients generally present to the physician with complaints of localized pain and stiffness. The pain may be related to specific muscle activity and may be progressive. It may eventually become chronic and result in a sleep disorder or chronic pain syndrome. Physical examination of the patient generally reveals local muscle pain. Trigger points may not be noted unless specifically sought. Knowledge of typical pain radiation patterns and trigger point locations is useful to the physician (Fig. 6.2). In our experience, MPS involving the shoulder and neck is most common, although it may involve any muscle.[13]

Management

Patients with MPS generally enjoy a good prognosis. The most critical elements of treatment include patient education and stretching of the involved muscle. Physical therapy may be useful for patient education, stretching instruction, and perhaps "spray and stretch," a procedure where a local vapocoolant spray is used over the involved area immediately before stretching. In resistant cases, injection of the trigger point with local anesthetic, followed immediately by stretching, can produce dramatic, prolonged relief. Multiple injections may be required. For some muscle groups, physical strengthening may help resolve the condition and help to prevent recurrence. MPS is less often associated with other medical conditions, including psychological conditions, than is FM. In MPS patients the use of biofeedback and relaxation therapy may help to teach them to discriminate between unnecessarily tense muscles and relaxed ones. Improved skills in dealing with life's stresses may be useful for treatment and prevention in these patients.

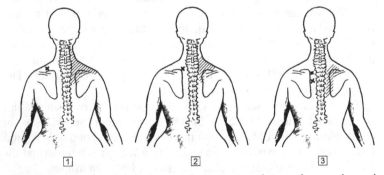

Fig. 6.2. Myofascial pain syndromes involving the neck and shoulder girdle. The involved muscles are (1) trapezius, (2) levator scapula, and (3) rhomboids. The distribution of pain is indicated by parallel lines, and the common trigger points are indicated by an X.

Complex Regional Pain Syndrome

Complex regional pain syndrome (CRPS) has replaced reflex sympathetic dystrophy (RSD) as the designation for a syndrome characterized by pain that is out of proportion to the inciting event, loss of function, and evidence of autonomic dysfunction. CRPS is subdivided into types I and II based on the nature of the initial injury. Cases of CRPS type I develop after nonspecific and often minor trauma to the affected area. Cases of CRPS type II evolve from definite injuries to peripheral nerves.[14]

Diagnosis

The clinical criteria[14] for diagnosis include the following: (1) diffuse pain, which is often nonanatomic and is frequently out of proportion to the initial injury; the pain may develop at any time relative to the injury; (2) loss of function, which can include any activity or motion impairment associated with the pain; and (3) sympathetic dysfunction, which includes some objective evidence of an autonomic dysfunction as represented by skin, soft tissue, or blood flow changes. It might also include atrophy of the skin or subcutaneous tissue, edema, Sudeck's osteoporosis, or a characteristic bone scan.

Complex regional pain syndrome usually has three phases: acute, dystrophic, and atrophic.[14] The *acute phase* is generally thought to be associated with signs of sympathetic denervation or underactivity, resulting in increased skin temperature, increased hair and nail growth, and edema. The acute phase usually lasts up to three months after the injury. The *dystrophic phase* is associated with hyperactivity of the sympathetic nervous system, which commonly translates into a burning pain, cold intolerance, cool skin, decreased hair and nail growth, hyperhidrosis, decreased range of motion, and atrophy. Behavioral and emotional changes are often seen during this phase and are often related to protecting the painful body part. The *atrophic phase* may be associated with decreased pain but is generally associated with irreversible changes in skin, subcutaneous tissue, and muscle. Fibrosis and contractures may develop. Testing helpful in documenting CRPS includes objective measurement of skin temperature (e.g., with thermography); measurement of blood flow (e.g., plethysmography or Doppler assessment); roentgenographic changes (e.g., with a three-phase bone scan or on plain radiographs); and response to neural blockade. Referral to an anesthesiologist for a trial of blockade, when accompanied by objective verification of a successful block and associated decrease in signs and symptoms, can be helpful from both diagnostic and treatment points of view.[15]

Management

Treatment of CRPS often requires multiple modalities and should not be associated with a further increase in pain or use of narcotics. For optimal effects, any treatment requires active participation of the patient. Effective treatment generally involves the following.

Physical Therapy. The early use of physical therapy is a mainstay of the successful treatment of patients with CRPS. Pain control can be enhanced through desensitization exercises and transcutaneous electrical nerve stimulator (TENS) units. Functional loss and atrophy can be minimized through exercises to mobilize and strengthen the affected area.[14]

Invasive Treatments. Chemical blockade, such as a stellate ganglion blockade or a regional Bier block, is often helpful early in the course of CRPS.[15] Multiple blocks may be required. Persistent cases have been treated with surgical sympathectomies and with implanted spinal cord electrical stimulators.[16]

Noninvasive Medications. A variety of medications has been used for CRPS,[17] but none is consistently effective, making treatment choices a largely empiric process. This inconsistency may represent varied pathophysiological mechanisms in CRPS. The most commonly used oral medications include NSAIDs for nonnarcotic pain relief, low-dose tricyclic antidepressants, and membrane-stabilizing anticonvulsants such as gabapentin.[14] Other medications that have resulted in some success include short-term use of corticosteroids, calcium channel blockers, α- and β-adrenergic antagonists, and intramuscular calcitonin. Useful topical regimens include lidocaine patches and capsaicin cream 0.025% applied four times daily to the affected area.[17]

Psychotherapy. It is important for the patient to maintain a positive emotional outlook, and psychotherapy directed to this goal may be useful. Additionally, therapy directed against some of the associated emotional consequences of CRPS may be useful, as anxiety, depression, and even suicide attempts are not uncommon in this group of patients.[17] Biofeedback is sometimes useful for dealing with CRPS.

Prevention

Although primary prevention is not possible for CRPS, secondary prevention is helpful. The earlier CRPS is diagnosed and treatment started, the better is the prognosis. Because psychological issues become more predominant the longer CRPS continues, addressing these issues early may also help minimize suffering and prevent suicide.

Family Issues

Family members may need help understanding why inconsequential trauma may cause such major problems. Including the family members in explanations may help ensure understanding and facilitate rapport, which is essential for treatment of this condition. Occasionally, the family, along with many healthcare professionals, views the symptoms of CRPS as somatization. Explanations to the family that CRPS is not primarily a psychological problem (but that it may have marked psychological implications) may help preserve family function.

Neuroma

A neuroma is a benign mass composed of disorganized axons and scar tissue. In any location it may cause pain but is especially sensitive when at a location that receives trauma or pressure. Neuromas commonly occur after trauma to a nerve or in the proximal portion of the nerve if it has been transected. The neuroma may form long after the initial nerve trauma. In the upper extremity, the most common locations for a neuroma are in the thumb (bowler's thumb) and the sensory branches of the radial nerve in the distal forearm. Treatment depends on the degree of symptoms, but it is not unusual for symptomatic neuromas of the upper extremities to require surgical excision. In the lower extremities, Morton's neuroma (MN) is the most common type. It represents an entrapment neuropathy of the interdigital nerve and is a common cause of forefoot pain, especially in women. The nerve is normally about 2 mm in diameter and generally does not cause symptoms until it reaches a size of 5 mm.[18]

Diagnosis

Morton's neuroma can usually be diagnosed clinically because of its characteristic sharp or burning pain on the plantar aspect of the foot, radiating to the tip of one or two toes. It most commonly involves the nerve in the third–fourth intermetatarsal space. The pain is usually made worse by walking, standing, or postures with the toes extended (e.g., standing on tiptoes). The physical findings include tenderness or reproduction of the pain when the interspace is compressed in a dorsoplantar or lateral direction. Numbness or tingling of the involved toes is common.

Management

This condition can often be managed through conservative means. Initially, a broad, soft shoe without elevated heels is used. A metatarsal bar support that removes pressure from the metatarsal head is also helpful. NSAIDs may also be useful. An orthotic device that stabilizes the foot in a neutral position is often helpful. Local injections of steroids may also be effective.[19] In cases that do not respond to conservative treatment, surgical resection of the neuroma (interdigital neurectomy), which leaves a residual numbness of the innervated toes, or release of the metatarsal ligament may be used. Approximately 80% of patients respond favorably to surgery.[20]

Prevention

The factor most conducive to prevention of MN is shoe selection. People should be encouraged to use a shoe wide enough to accommodate the foot comfortably and to avoid high-heeled shoes.

Dupuytren's Contracture

Dupuytren's contracture (DC) is a disease of the palmar and digital fascia characterized by a progressive fibrosis of the palmar aponeurosis, resulting in a flexion deformity of the fingers. The condition is most common in white-skinned races, especially those of Celtic origin.[21] It is two to seven times more common in men than women. It is seen most commonly between the ages of 50 and 70 years. DC is commonly seen in association with alcoholism, hyperlipidemia, epilepsy, and diabetes. One researcher found a 40% co-occurrence between Dupuytren's and epilepsy.[22] This connection is thought to be due to the genetic transmission common to the two conditions. In another study, DC was noted in 42% of 150 diabetics, compared to 18% of a control group.[23] This association is strong enough that physicians need to be vigilant about diagnosing diabetes when treating patients with DC (see Reference 33, Chapter 120). The pathognomonic sign of DC is a nodule in the palm, usually located at the base of the ring finger. The other fingers or thumb may also be involved but less commonly than the ring finger. This nodule may be painful or pruritic. The right hand is more commonly affected (regardless of hand dominance), but the condition is bilateral about half of the time. The diagnosis is usually easy and is made by palpating a characteristic nodule or cord in the typical palmar location (Fig. 6.3). If left untreated, the flexion contracture progresses. There are no proved nonsurgical methods for treating DC.[21] No one surgical technique has been found that is universally effective, but some type of fasciotomy

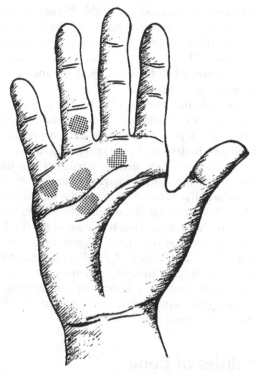

Fig. 6.3. Characteristic sites of palmar nodules (stippled areas) of Dupuytren's contracture. The right hand is more commonly involved, regardless of hand dominance.

is generally required. The optimal timing of surgical therapy is also not clear, but most authors recommend surgery when the metacarpophalangeal (MCP) joint contracture reaches 30 degrees or more. After surgery, the recurrence rate is about 50% if the patients are followed up for at least five years.[24]

Ganglion Cysts

Ganglion cysts, which are common benign tumors, may arise from a joint capsule or the synovial sheath of a tendon. They may maintain their connection to the synovial sheath or joint, in which case they may vary in size. The dorsal or volar wrist is the region where most ganglia occur. Ganglia may occur at any age but are most commonly seen between the ages of 20 and 40 and in women.[25] Ganglia may be obvious or occult. With occult cysts, patients may complain of a dull ache and tenderness, but no mass is palpable.[26] They may become evident by causing a compression neuropathy or compartment syndrome. This condition should be kept in mind when wrist pain of unknown etiology is encountered. Magnetic resonance imaging (MRI) or ultrasound techniques may be helpful in assessing the anatomy of the wrist when an occult cyst is suspected.

With obvious cysts the onset is usually insidious, although some patients report a history of acute onset associated with heavy use or trauma. Patients may report weakness or altered range of motion of the wrists or fingers. Radiation of pain into the forearm is not unusual. The examination reveals a firm, usually nontender cyst that feels like a small marble under the skin. A characteristic history and physical examination are usually sufficient to make the diagnosis, but aspiration of jellylike fluid confirms the diagnosis. A large-bore needle is usually required because of the viscous nature of the fluid. Instillation of steroids into the cyst may be helpful. If patients are symptomatic or if the appearance is unacceptable to the patient, surgical removal is the treatment of choice. When counseling patients or assessing the effectiveness of treatment, one must remember that approximately half of these cysts disappear without therapy[26] and that regardless of therapy recurrence is common.

Abnormalities of Bone

Benign Tumors

The primary care physician refers most of the patients found to have tumors involving bone, but it is helpful to have some understanding of these conditions in order to have a better idea of what to expect for the patient. No one system of classification is entirely satisfactory for all tumors, and a comprehensive inclusion of all types of tumors is beyond the scope of this chapter. Thus only the most common representatives of bone-related problems are discussed: benign tumors, neoplastic tumors, and miscellaneous problems.

Osteochondroma

Osteochondroma, also called exostosis, may be thought of as a developmental aberration of epiphyseal bone growth.[27] Bony projections, covered with cartilage caps, are found. Males are affected three times more commonly than females. The lesions are often single but can be part of a hereditary condition called osteochondromatosis. The lesions occur most commonly in the long bones of the extremities. They occasionally result in derangement of epiphyseal growth, causing bowing or shortening of the bones. Growth of the osteochondroma usually stops at the time of epiphyseal closure.

Osteoma

Osteomas are benign projections of densely sclerotic bone from cortical surfaces, usually the facial bones or skull.[27] They may arise at any age and are usually of little clinical significance unless they obstruct a sinus, impinge on the brain, or cause some cosmetic concern. They do not tend to transform into other types of lesions and do not usually require treatment unless they cause symptoms.

Osteoid Osteoma

Osteoid osteomas are usually found in young adults. They are twice as common in males as females. They are usually painful, which prompts the patient to seek medical help. The pain is usually nocturnal and dramatically responsive to aspirin. They are usually located at the ends of the tibia and femur. They appear as small radiolucent foci surrounded by densely sclerotic bone (Fig. 6.4). They can usually be managed by local excision.[28] When the lesions are larger than 2 cm in greatest dimension, they are, by definition, osteoblastomas.

Chondroma

Chondromas are composed of mature hyaline cartilage. They frequently arise within the interior of a bone and so are called enchondromas. They occur singly in either sex and most commonly between the ages of 20 and 50. There are genetic conditions where these tumors occur multiply, the most common of which is Ollier's disease. With the single chondroma, transformation into a sarcoma is rare. Most of the single lesions occur in the small bones of the hands or feet. Most of the lesions are asymptomatic and may be noticed incidentally or by some bone deformation. They rarely result in pain through pathologic fracture. Excision of the lesions may be required to exclude the possibility of chondrosarcoma,[27] a rare transformation except in individuals with Ollier's disease, where multiple enchondromas are seen.

Giant Cell Tumor

A relatively rare lesion, the giant cell tumor is most commonly seen in individuals between the ages of 20 and 50. Patients usually present with local pain or functional dysfunction related to the location of the tumor. About half of these tumors occur in the knee. Radiographs reveal the typical, large lytic "soap-bubble" lesions. The cell of origin of these tumors is not clear, and the biological behavior is somewhat

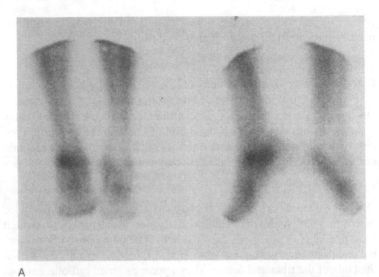

A

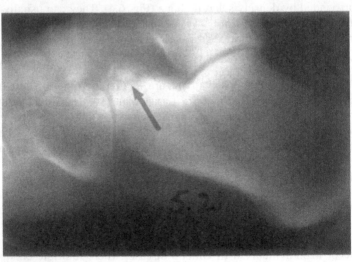

B

Fig. 6.4. Young woman with persistent foot pain and normal plain films of the foot. (A) Bone scan revealed a focus of uptake. (B) Tomography confirmed the presence of an osteoid osteoma (arrow).

erratic. Although most of these tumors are benign, they may be aggressive, eroding into the joint space and surrounding tissues. Treatment is usually conservative, with curettage or conservative resection. However, after treatment, the tumors commonly recur, although it may be years later. Up to 4% of these tumors metastasize to the lungs, usually after surgical resection.[27]

Malignant Bone Tumors

Malignant tumors of bone may originate in the bone or metastasize to the bone. There are definite patterns in tumor type based on the age of the patient.

Ewing's Sarcoma

Ewing's sarcoma is a tumor of uncertain origin. It is most common in children and young adults. It is more common in whites than blacks. The tumor may occur in any bone but has some predilection for long tubular bones and the pelvis. The presenting complaints include pain, swelling, tenderness, and erythema, which makes it resemble osteomyelitis. Early there may be no radiographic abnormalities, but later a typical lytic lesion with an "onion-skin" appearance of the periosteum is seen. The prognosis is improving with the use of surgery, chemotherapy, and in some cases radiotherapy. Long-term cures are now seen in about 50% of five-year survivors.[27]

Primary Chondrosarcoma

A cartilage-producing bone tumor, primary chondrosarcoma occurs most commonly during middle to late life. It occurs most commonly in the central skeleton. The tumors are slow-growing and late in metastasizing, resulting in a relatively favorable prognosis. They are graded on the basis of anaplasia, and most of the tumors fall into the low anaplastic categories.[27] Because they are slow-growing, patients may present with a bony mass that has been present for years. Radiographs demonstrate radiolucent lesions with increased uptake on bone scintigraphy.[29] Successful treatment requires total removal of the tumor. The specimen's pathological analysis has prognostic value, with the lower grades of anaplasia being associated with a higher five-year survival.

Osteosarcoma

Osteosarcoma is an aggressive tumor of mesenchymal cell origin characterized by formation of bone by the tumor. Except for myeloma, it is the most common primary bone cancer. These tumors can generally be split into primary and secondary types. Primary osteosarcomas occur most commonly in children and young adults and are most common in males. There appears to be a genetic predisposition. The secondary osteosarcomas generally develop in adults in areas of abnormal bone (e.g., Paget's disease) or in response to some sort of carcinogen exposure (most commonly irradiation). The most common presenting complaints of patients with osteosarcoma are local pain, tenderness, and swelling. It most often occurs in the medullary cavity of the metaphyseal end of the long bones of the extremities. Radiographs, computed tomography (CT) scans, or MRI scans often provide a characteristic picture of subperiosteal or soft tissue penetration of the tumor with extraosseous bone density. To confirm the diagnosis, however, biopsy is required. Great advances have been made in treatment recently, with a combination of surgery, radiotherapy, and chemotherapy (depending on the specific type of lesion) providing the best chances for survival.[27]

Chordoma

Chordoma is a malignant bone tumor seen most commonly in the sacrum and spine. It is thought to arise from remnants of the notochord. These tumors are usually seen in middle-aged and elderly adults. Radiographs, CT scans, or MRI scans usually show the mixed lytic and sclerotic lesions of the chordoma.[30]

Metastatic Malignant Tumors

Tumors that commonly metastasize to bone include thyroid, breast, prostate, bronchus, kidney, bladder, uterus, ovary, testicle, and adrenal tumors. Lymphomas most commonly spread to bone from primary involvement of lymph nodes but also are seen rarely primarily in the skeleton. Bone scans are thought to be the best screening test for patients suspected of having skeletal metastasis.[31] Patients with metastatic bone disease most often present with pathological fracture or pain. The radiographical appearance of these lesions tends to be sclerotic in prostate and breast metastasis and lytic in lung, bowel, kidney, and thyroid. Biopsy of the bony lesion is helpful for determining whether the lesion is metastatic.

Miscellaneous Bone Conditions

Nonossifying Fibroma

A common condition, nonossifying fibroma is also called a fibrous cortical defect. It is considered a developmental aberration rather than a neoplasm. It is seen primarily in children and occurs most commonly in the femur, tibia, and fibula. The diagnosis can usually be made by the radiographic picture, and a large number of these lesions are found while obtaining a radiograph for another purpose. The lesions are sharply demarcated, lobular, radiolucent defects in the metaphyseal cortex. There is often an intact, thin layer of subperiosteal cortical bone. The lesions may range in size from a few millimeters to 5 cm. They are usually asymptomatic and are seen in approximately one third of children.[27] The larger lesions may cause pain and predispose the child to fracture. These lesions do not tend to transform into neoplasms and often disappear spontaneously.

Paget's Disease of Bone

Osteitis deformans (Paget's disease of bone) is characterized by excessive bone destruction and disorganized repair, resulting in mottled increased density and bony deformity.[27] There is a genetic component to this lesion, although many people develop clinically insignificant lesions. The condition is thought to be related to a canine distemper (paramyxovirus) infection.[32]

Diagnosis. Paget's disease is often asymptomatic and discovered incidentally by radiography. When symptomatic, nighttime bone pain is usually the first symptom. Because of bone softening, bowing of the tibias, pathological fractures, and increased kyphosis are commonly seen. An increasing head circumference, deafness, and a waddling gait are other relatively common symptoms. A markedly elevated serum alkaline phosphatase level and normal calcium and phosphorus are the usual laboratory pattern. An elevated 24-hour urinary hydroxyproline level, indicative of rapid bone turnover, is also seen. Radiographic findings include expanded bone with increased density. Early on, radiolucent lesions are common, especially in the skull and pelvis (Fig. 6.5). Later mixed, then sclerotic lesions are seen.[27] A bone scan can detect lesions before they become apparent on plain radiographs.

Complications. The complications of Paget's disease include fractures, spinal cord compression, malignant degeneration, and hypercalcemia-related problems such as renal stones. The latter complication is seen primarily if there is excessive calcium intake along with immobilization.

Treatment. Treatment is warranted only if significant symptoms are present. NSAIDs can be of value in suppressing bone activity and controlling mild symptoms. Calcitonins and diphosphonates suppress

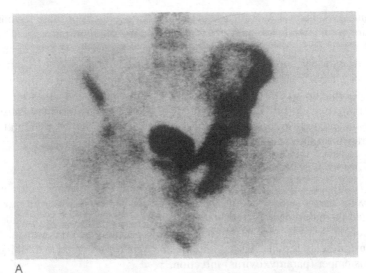

A

B

Fig. 6.5. (A) Bone scan shows extensive uptake in half of the pelvis in this patient with nocturnal pelvic pain. (B) Plain film shows coarse trabeculae over the acetabulum (black arrow) and a thickening of the iliopectineal line (white arrow), findings seen with Paget's disease.

bone resorption mediated by osteoclasts and are effective in Paget's disease. These treatments have significant potential side effects and complications. The alkaline phosphatase level can be used to monitor disease activity.

Prognosis. The later in life that Paget's disease begins, the better is the prognosis. The progression is usually slow, over years. Renal complications and malignant degeneration of lesions are associated with a poor prognosis.

References

1. Clauw DJ. Fibromyalgia: More than just a musculoskeletal disease. *Am Fam Physician.* 1995;52:843–51.
2. Goldenberg DL. Fibromyalgia syndrome: An emerging but controversial condition. *JAMA.* 1987;257:2782–7.
3. Stormorken H, Brosstad F. Fibromyalgia: Family clustering and sensory urgency with early onset indicate genetic predisposition and thus a "true" disease [letter]. *Scand J Rheumatol.* 1992;21:207–11.
4. Silman A, Schollum J, Croft P. The epidemiology of tender point counts in the general population [abstract]. *Arthritis Rheum.* 1993;36(suppl):48.
5. Granges G, Littlejohn GO. A comparative study of clinical signs in fibromyalgia/fibrositis syndrome, healthy and exercising subjects. *J Rheumatol.* 1993;20:344–51.
6. Reynolds WJ, Moldofsky H, Saskin P, et al. The effects of cyclobenzaprine on sleep physiology and symptoms in patients with fibromyalgia. *J Rheumatol.* 1991;18:452–4.
7. Simms RW, Goldenberg DL. Symptoms mimicking neurologic disorders in fibromyalgia syndrome. *J Rheumatol.* 1988;15:1271–3.
8. Pellegrino MJ, Van Fossen D, Gordon C, et al. Prevalence of mitral valve prolapse in primary fibromyalgia: A pilot investigation. *Arch Phys Med Rehabil.* 1989;70:541–3.
9. Goldenberg DL. Management of fibromyalgia syndrome. *Rheum Dis Clin North Am.* 1989;15:499–512.
10. Felson DT, Goldenberg DL. The natural history of fibromyalgia. *Arthritis Rheum.* 1986;29:1522–6.
11. Yunus MB, Kalyan-Raman UP, Kalyan-Raman K. Primary fibromyalgia syndrome and myofascial pain syndrome: Clinical features and muscle pathology. *Arch Phys Med Rehabil.* 1988;69:451–4.
12. Thompson JM. Tension myalgia as a diagnosis at the Mayo Clinic and its relationship to fibrositis, fibromyalgia, and myofascial pain syndrome. *Mayo Clin Proc.* 1990;65:1237–48.
13. Harden RN, Bruehl SP, Gass S, Niemiec C, Barbick B. Signs and symptoms of the myofascial pain syndrome: A national survey of pain management providers. *Clin J Pain.* 2000;16(1):64–72.
14. Lederhaas G. Complex regional pain syndrome: New emphasis. *Emerg Med.* 2000;32:18–22.

15. Warfield CA. The sympathetic dystrophies. *Hosp Pract.* 1984;May: 52c–j.
16. Kemler MA, Barendse GAM, Kleef M, et al. Spinal cord stimulation with chronic reflex sympathetic dystrophy. *N Engl J Med.* 2000;343(9):618–24.
17. Haddox JD, Van Alstine D. Pharmacologic therapy for reflex sympathetic dystrophy. *Phys Med Rehabil.* 1996;10:297–309.
18. Redd RA, Peters VJ, Emery SF, et al. Morton neuroma: Sonographic evaluation. *Radiology.* 1989;171:415–17.
19. Strong G, Thomas PS. Conservative treatment of Morton's neuroma. *Orthop Rev.* 1987;16:343–5.
20. Mann RA. Pain in the foot. 2. Causes of pain in the hindfoot, midfoot, and forefoot. *Postgrad Med.* 1987;82:167–74.
21. Riolo J, Young VL, Ueda K, et al. Dupuytren's contracture. *South Med J.* 1991;84:983–96.
22. James JIP. The relationship of Dupuytren's contracture and epilepsy. *Hand.* 1969;1:47–9.
23. Noble J, Heathcote JG, Cohen H. Diabetes mellitus in the aetiology of Dupuytren's disease. *J Bone Joint Surg.* 1984;66B:322–5.
24. McFarlane RM. The current status of Dupuytren's disease. *J Hand Surg.* 1983;8:703–8.
25. Smith DL, Wernick R. Common nonarticular syndromes in the elbow, wrist, and hand. *Postgrad Med.* 1994;95:173–91.
26. Jennings CD. Deciding whether and how to treat painful ganglia. *J Musculoskel Med.* 1986;3:39–46.
27. Rosenberg AE. Skeletal system and soft tissue tumors. In: Cotran RS, Kumar V, Robbins SL, eds. *Robbins' Pathologic Basis of Disease.* Philadelphia: Saunders, 1994;1213–46.
28. Healey JH, Ghelan B. Osteoid osteoma and osteoblastoma. *Clin Orthop.* 1986;204:76–85.
29. Vande Streek PR, Carretta RF, Weiland FL. Nuclear medicine approaches to musculoskeletal disease. *Radiol Clin North Am.* 1994;32:227–53.
30. Tumors and infiltrative lesions of the lumbosacral spine. In: Borenstein DG, Wiesel SW, Boden SD, eds. *Low Back Pain.* Philadelphia: Saunders, 1995;390–5.
31. Ell PJ. Bones and joints. In: Maisey MN, Britton KE, Gilday DL, eds. *Clinical Nuclear Medicine.* Philadelphia: Saunders, 1983;135–65.
32. Cartwright EJ, Gordon MT, Freemont AJ, et al. Paramyxoviruses and Paget's disease. *J Med Virol.* 1993;40:133–41.
33. Taylor RB, ed. *Family Medicine: Principles and Practice.* 6th ed. New York: Springer, 2003.

7
Musculoskeletal Problems of Children

Mark D. Bracker, Suraj A. Achar, Todd J. May, Juan Carlos Buller, and Wilma J. Wooten

Torsional and Other Variations of the Lower Extremity

Gait Abnormalities

Rotational problems resulting in gait abnormalities are the most common orthopedic conditions in the pediatric age group. Parents are frequently concerned that their child will grow up deformed or be unable to play sports as they observe in-toeing or out-toeing and seek medical attention. Recent studies, however, have shown athletes with internal tibial torsion are faster than age-matched controls.[1] Most rotational abnormalities resolve spontaneously as musculature develops, and knowing this fact is reassuring to parents. Rarely, conditions remain fixed and require surgical correction at an older age. Torsional deformities may be due to problems in the foot (metatarsus adductus), tibia (torsion), or femur and hip (femoral anteversion). Angular abnormalities (bowlegs, knock-knees) generally resolve spontaneously as well. Certain terminology has been recommended as well as specific testing used to evaluate gait (Fig. 7.1).

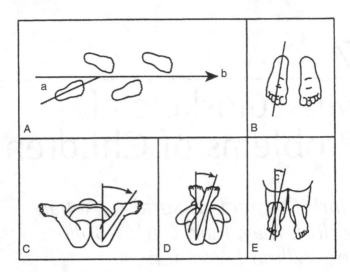

Fig. 7.1. Tests for torsional deformities (see text for full discussion). (A) Foot progression angle (a) is formed by the foot axis (B) and the line of progression (b). (B) Foot axis. (C) Measurement of internal femoral rotation. (D) Measurement of external femoral rotation. (E) Thigh-foot angle (c) is formed by the longitudinal axis of the femur and the foot axis. (From Lillegard and Kruse,[50] with permission.)

Terminology

Definitions of the terms used in this chapter are as follows.

Angle of gait (foot progression angle): Angle of the intersection between the foot axis and the line progression. It is the result of static and dynamic influences from the foot to the hip. This angle remains relatively stable at 8 to 12 degrees of out-toeing through growth. There is a wide range of normal values varying from 3 degrees in-toeing to 20 degrees out-toeing; in one study of 130 children, 4.5% had an in-toeing gait.[2] Abnormalities anywhere along this kinetic chain (including hip, leg, and foot) can change the angle of gait.

Femoral antetorsion: Anteversion beyond the normal range [2 standard deviations (SD)].

Femoral anteversion: Angular difference between the forward inclination of the femoral neck and the transcondylar femoral axis (Fig. 7.2).

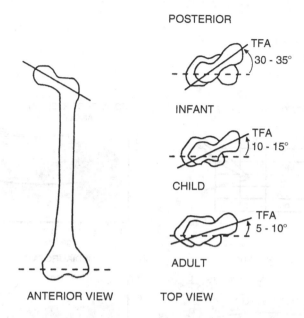

Fig. 7.2. Transcondylar femoral axis (TFA) as it would be measured radiographically in degrees of rotation.

Foot axis: Imaginary line bisecting the long axis of the foot from the mid-heel through the middle to the metatarsal heads.

Internal and external femoral rotation: The child lies prone with the knees flexed to 90 degrees, the pelvis is stabilized, and the angle of gravity-assisted internal (medial rotation) and external rotation (lateral rotation) of each leg is measured.

Thigh–foot angle: Measures tibial torsion. The child lies prone and flexes the knees to 90 degrees; the angle is then placed in neutral position. Looking down at the sole of the foot, an imaginary line through the long axis of the foot is measured against the long axis of the femur. The angle between these two axes is the thigh–foot angle.

Evaluation and Interpretation

The medical history is obtained first and includes the type of deformity, apparent time of onset, amount of progression, family history, and previous treatment. A complete musculoskeletal and neurological examination is performed, and finally a torsional (rotational) profile is generated to determine the severity and level of deformity (Fig. 7.3).

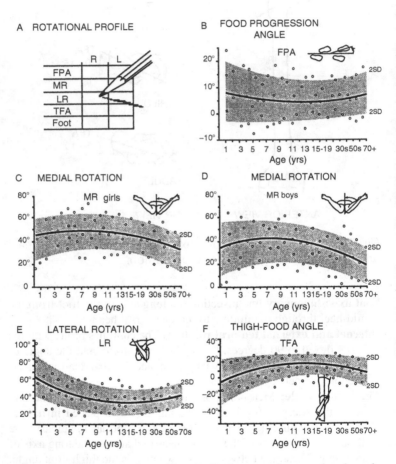

Fig. 7.3. (A) Torsional profile. (B–F) Range of normal values by age group and sex. (From Engel and Staheli,[2] with permission.)

Foot Progression Angle. It is important to watch the child walk as naturally as possible. When being observed, children may initially try to control the amount of in-toeing to please the parent or physician. Keep in mind also that the amount of in-toeing becomes worse when a child is fatigued. In-toeing is expressed as a negative value (12–10 degrees) and out-toeing as a positive value. The normal value range for the foot progression angle is wide, and severe deformity above the foot may exist with a normal angle.

Hip Rotation. With the child in the prone position, the knees are flexed to 90 degrees with the pelvis level. The thigh is then rotated medially (internal rotation of the hip) by gravity alone. Lateral rotation is measured with the child in the same position by allowing the legs to cross. The diagnosis of medial femoral torsional deformity/ femoral anteversion is made if medial rotation is more than 70 degrees. Total joint laxity must be taken into consideration by concurrent reduction in lateral rotation. Restriction of lateral rotation during early infancy is thought to be due to intrauterine position.

Tibial Rotation. Tibial rotation, the most difficult measurement to make accurately, requires assessment of the thigh–foot angle (TFA). The TFA increases from early childhood to mid-childhood. Internal tibial rotation is expressed as a negative angle. A negative value up to 20 degrees is considered normal during infancy. Medial tibial torsion exists if the TFA is more than 20 degrees. During early childhood the tibia rotates laterally.

Foot. The sole of the foot is observed to determine its shape; the lateral border is normally straight. Metatarsus adductus is the characteristic appearance of a "bean-shaped foot" with a wide space between the first and second toes, prominence at the base of the fifth metatarsal bone, and convexity at the lateral side of the foot. Metatarsus adductus is often present in conjunction with tibial torsion.

Clinical Patterns and Management

In-toeing (Metatarsus Adductus). The terms *metatarsus adductus* (MA) and *metatarsus varus* are used interchangeably. MA occurs when the forefoot bones are deviated medially at the tarsal–metatarsal junction, causing the foot to appear to curve inward at the midfoot (bean-shaped foot). It is probably caused by a combination of intrauterine position and genetic predisposition and can be either flexible or rigid. Studies dispute the belief that hip dysplasia is higher among patients with metatarsus varus than in the general population.[3] On physical examination the foot is convex laterally and concave medially. The lateral border of the base of the fifth metatarsal may appear prominent. With the heel held in neutral position and pressure directed laterally at the first metatarsal head, a flexible deformity corrects to neutral but does not overcorrect as do normal feet. One helpful test is to stroke the lateral border of the foot, noting if the infant reflexively corrects the deformity. Treatment for flexible MA involves having the parents passively correct the range of deformity (as described above) with each diaper change. Due to the high rate of spontaneous resolution and the history of natural resolution, no treatment has been shown to be superior. These treatments vary from observation to casting to bracing night or day, or both, to orthopedic shoes. Children with rigid MA require cast correction and are best treated before 6 months of age and worked up for other neuromuscular disorders. If begun during the first month of life, correction can often be obtained within 6 to 8 weeks of casting by a knowledgeable orthopedist. After age 8 months, cast correction is almost impossible due to foot stiffness and active kicking by robust toddlers.

The reasons for treating these feet remain controversial, and specific treatment indications vary among orthopedic surgeons. It is currently believed that residual MA is not linked to adult degenerative arthritis.[1] Surgical correction is rarely indicated. When needed, Heyman–Herndon soft tissue releases are advised for children under age 4 years, and multiple metatarsal osteotomies are recommended for older children.[4] In severe cases requiring surgical correction, associated heel valgus is common and must be addressed or the child will be further disabled because correction of the forefoot alone removes the stable tripod of the foot.

Tibial Torsion. In-toeing can also be due to excessive internal tibial torsion (medial tibial version). It can be clinically estimated using the TFA described previously. Normally the tibia is externally rotated 5 degrees at birth and 15 degrees at skeletal maturity. Correction is almost always spontaneous. Bracing, splints, twister cables, and shoe modifications have not been shown to be effective and are not recommended, as most of these deformities correct spontaneously by 3 to 4 years of age.[5] Developmental correction may be delayed if the child sleeps prone with the legs internally rotated or sits with the knees flexed and feet internally rotated. Although there is no proved benefit of altering the child's sitting position, parents may be instructed to encourage the child to avoid these positions. Derotational osteotomy is reserved for severe deformity, including significant functional and cosmetic disability, internal rotation of more than 85 degrees, external rotation of less than 10 degrees, radiographic anteversion of more than 45 degrees, or external tibial rotation of less than 35 degrees. The child must be at least 7 to 8 years old.[6]

Femoral Anteversion. The angle between the femoral neck axis and the transcondylar axis of the distal femur is called femoral version (Fig. 7.2). Femoral anteversion (FA) decreases from an average of 40 degrees at birth to about 15 degrees at skeletal maturity. Children commonly sit on their knees with their feet out to the sides in the classic W position. With femoral anteversion the in-toeing is worse at the end of the day when compensating muscles fatigue. FA presents by age 3 to 4 years and resolves slowly over the next 5 years and is more common in girls than boys.

Infants normally have limited medial rotation due to a tight hip capsule, and external rotation to 90 degrees is common. External rotation decreases to around 55 degrees by age 3 and slowly decreases thereafter. Internal rotation increases from 35 degrees at birth to 60 degrees by age 6, at which time it is slightly greater than external rotation. From birth to 2 years of age the total range should be 120 degrees, decreasing to 95 to 110 degrees thereafter.

Treatment for an in-toeing gait due to excessive femoral anteversion, termed medial femoral torsion, is almost always simple observation, as 85% resolve with spontaneous derotation of the proximal femur during normal growth. Bony derotation occurs up to age 8 and in some cases into adolescence. Surgery is rarely indicated; it is reserved for severe, uncompensated medial femoral torsion causing significant functional and cosmetic problems during late childhood. In rare severe cases, a proximal femoral derotation osteotomy can be done safely at age 9 or 10.

Angular Abnormalities of the Knee

Newborns generally have a genu varus of approximately 15 degrees due physiologically to intrauterine positioning. Parents frequently note bowed legs as their child starts to stand. Children with superimposed internal tibial torsion actually look more bowed than they are. Children progress from genu varus in the newborn until 24 months and then start to develop genu valgus to about 15 degrees by age 4 years. Then by 6 to 7 years of age, this valgus begins to correct to 5 to 6 degrees, where it essentially remains to adulthood. Pathologic genu valgum or varus should be evaluated for metabolic disorders, inflammatory disease, tumors, osteochondrodysplasia, posttraumatic conditions, congenital abnormalities, osteogenesis imperfecta, or Blount's disease as possible causes.

Bowlegs

Excessive genu varus deformities with a tibial–femoral angle of more than 20 degrees should be investigated if they have not started correcting by 2 years of age. Growth charts should be carefully reviewed along with developmental and family history. Evaluation should include physical exam, gait observation, knee ligament laxity assessment, rotational evaluation, and foot position. Appropriate laboratory and standing radiographic studies should be ordered. The posteroanterior (PA) standing radiographs must be taken with the child's feet together or a shoulder width apart and neutral rotation with the patella pointing directly forward. The physis should be carefully examined. A tibiofemoral angle of more than 20 degrees in toddlers indicates severe physiologic bowing, or Blount's disease. Severe physiologic bowing is characterized radiographically as follows.

1. Medial metaphyseal beaking of the proximal fibula and distal femur
2. Medial cortical thickening
3. Varus angulation of more than 20 degrees based on the metaphyseal–diaphyseal angle
4. No pathologic changes in the proximal tibial epiphysis

After other etiologies have been ruled out and severe physiologic bowing is diagnosed, spontaneous correction can be expected by 7 to 8 years of age. If significant deformity persists past age 8, corrective tibial osteotomy is necessary in certain cases.

Blount's Disease

Osteochondrosis deformans tibiae, or Blount's disease, is due to defective formation of the posterior medial border of the proximal tibial epiphysis and may be difficult to distinguish from severe physiologic bowing. Blount's disease is more common in blacks than whites and is associated with obesity and early walking. Radiographic findings after 18 to 24 months are angulation under the posterior medial proximal epiphysis, metaphyseal irregularity, beaking of the proximal tibia, and wedging of the proximal epiphysis. Another radiographic sign that has been found useful to diagnose Blount's disease is the metaphyseal–diaphyseal (MD) angle. The angle is derived from drawing a line along the lateral tibial cortex on a standard PA radiograph, and then drawing a line perpendicular to the tibial cortex line and one through the epiphysis. If the angle between the epiphysis and tibial cortex perpendicular line is greater than 11 degrees, Blount's disease is diagnosed.[7] Most of these children require corrective bracing or surgery and should be referred as soon as identified.

Knock-Knees

Genu valgus (knock-knees) can be apparent, physiologic, or pathologic. Apparent valgus may be due to large thighs, joint laxity, or poor muscle tone. Most cases are idiopathic or physiologic. Pathologic causes include juvenile rheumatoid arthritis, rickets, trauma, endocrine disturbance, and infection. Most children have a slight genu valgus that generally resolves by 6 years of age; it can become excessive later during childhood or early adolescence when the normal valgus fails to resolve. Genu valgus may represent an acceleration of normal angulation caused by abnormal forces across the knee. Standing PA radiographs with the feet pointing straight ahead may be obtained to document the tibiofemoral angle and to rule out underlying disease. Young children with this problem tend toward spontaneous resolution. With older children, knock-knees is less likely to correct completely.

Surgical correction of severe knock-knees deformity causing significant functional or cosmetic problems should be performed 1 year before the end of physeal growth in the femur (girls, 10–11 years old; boys, 12–13 years old). A staple encircles the femoral physis, which continues to grow laterally but not medially.[8]

Problems of the Feet

Toe Walking

The tiptoe gait characteristic of beginning toddlers should give way to an adult-like pattern by 2 years of age. Neuromuscular conditions such as cerebral palsy or spinal cord lesions such as spina bifida, tethered cord, and diastematomyelia can produce foot deformity, which can be appropriately evaluated diagnostically or referral made if toe walking persists beyond age 2.

Clubfoot

Talipes equinovarus (clubfoot), which occurs in approximately 1/1000 births,[9] is characterized by talar plantar flexion, hindfoot varus, forefoot adduction, and soft tissue contractures, resulting in a cavus foot deformity (Fig. 7.4).[10] It is thought to be secondary to intrauterine position in a genetically predisposed fetus but is also associated with congenital hip dislocation, myelomeningocele, and arthrogryposis. The major deformity of clubfoot is in the subtalar complex, with shortening and medial deviation of the talus with displacement of the navicular medially.[11] Radiographs confirm the severity of deformity, allow comparisons over time, and are essential for judging the type of surgical correction needed.

Treatment by an experienced orthopedic surgeon is an acquired skill that is becoming a lost art. Proper intervention involves reduction of the displaced navicular on the head of the talus and mobilization of tight capsules and tendons through manipulation followed by placement in a series of carefully molded corrective casts. The need for extensive surgery is reduced if casting is early and effective with 30% to 50% correction obtained.[12] Operative intervention is indicated if complete correction cannot be obtained or maintained. Recognition and treatment of clubfoot deformity should be initiated in the newborn nursery; therefore, recognition and referral of this entity are imperative. Parents should be reassured it is normal for the affected foot and calf to be smaller throughout the child's life.

Cavus Foot

Pes cavus, or cavus foot, is a fixed equinus and pronation deformity of the forefoot in relation to the hindfoot, usually resulting from an

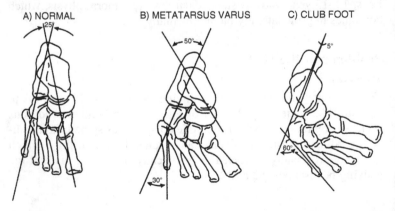

Fig. 7.4. Bone alignment. (A) Normal foot. (B) Metatarsus adductus (varus). (C) Clubfoot, demonstrating Kite's angle. Note Kite's angle is increased in metatarsus varus and decreased in club foot.

underlying neuromuscular condition: spinal dysraphism (spina bifida, lipoma, tethered cord, diastematomyelia), Charcot–Marie–Tooth disease, Friedreich's ataxia, or cord tumor. Occasionally, cases are familial or idiopathic. When unilateral, a spinal disorder is almost always the cause. All cavus feet demonstrate excessive plantar flexion of the first ray with pronation of the forefoot in relation to the hindfoot. The workup includes family and neurological history and exam, weight-bearing radiographs of the feet, and strong consideration of a referral to the orthopedist. Corrective shoes and inserts are not effective for treating cavus feet. Surgical management, best undertaken after age 4 or 5 years, is directed toward medial and plantar release (plantar fascia, short flexors, adductor hallucis) followed by weekly cast changes to gain full correction.[13]

Flatfoot

Flexible Flatfoot

All children have flat feet at birth. Some of these feet remain flat and asymptomatic and are a normal physiologic variant. The normal foot may appear flat until the child is 3 to 5 years old. Reasons include ligament laxity, flexibility of cartilage, neuromuscular development, and the presence of subcutaneous fat that occupies space in the arch. The support ligaments gradually tighten to form the longitudinal arch, increasing definition with normal growth. As a result, the true flexible flatfoot is difficult to diagnose clinically before the child is 2 years old.

The cause is primarily laxity of the ligaments that normally support the bones forming the arch. The laxity is frequently familial and is sometimes associated with Down, Marfan, and Ehlers–Danlos syndromes, all of which include excessive ligament laxity. Testing is done by having the child dorsiflex the great toe or stand on tiptoe (looking for the formation of an arch). Observed from the rear, the patient may have calcaneal valgus when bearing weight, shifting to varus position when standing tiptoe (a reflection of subtalar flexibility).[14]

Radiographic evaluation aids in confirming the diagnosis, localizing the malaligned joints, and ruling out other possibilities in the differential diagnosis. Anteroposterior and lateral radiographs are obtained with the patient standing so the feet are in the weight-bearing position.

No treatment is necessary for the asymptomatic foot, as there is gradual improvement with growth and development; the greatest improvement is seen by age 4. Recent studies have shown no greater incidence of painful adult feet in children with flexible flat feet.[12] The use of arch supports in asymptomatic children with flexible flatfoot has not been shown to make a difference in terms of altering the radiographic or clinical outcome.[14] For the occasional child who does develop a symptomatic flexible flatfoot, correction with an orthosis may be indicated. Medial longitudinal arch supports are helpful, and a medial heel wedge is added if calcaneal valgus is present.

Rigid Flatfoot

A rigid flatfoot is flat both sitting and standing; it may be due to underlying conditions such as infection, old trauma, congenital vertical talus, or tarsal coalition. Rigid pes planus with normal (nonspastic) peroneals is usually caused by an old infection of the tarsus, rheumatoid arthritis, or injury resulting in ankylosis and deformity that persists after the symptoms of the original pathology have subsided.[15] Rigid pes planus with associated spasm of the peroneus muscles, termed peroneal spastic flatfoot, is most often secondary to tarsal coalition or less commonly tarsal joint arthritis, tuberculosis, or old trauma. The decreased range of motion is due primarily to ankylosis, and the peroneal spasm is probably secondary to stress from the rigid tarsus. This stress results in painful strains, which initiate reflux muscle spasms of the peroneals.[15] Deformity of the foot secondary to cerebral palsy is common. Typically, the spastic flatfoot occurs in an ambulatory diplegic individual. In this case contracture of the Achilles tendon is the primary problem. Tarsal coalitions may be identified on plain radiographs but are often cartilaginous and best identified with a computed tomography (CT) scan. Orthopedic surgeons must exercise care regarding patient selection for surgery. All foot surgery is characterized by several weeks to months of disability during the postoperative period. The adolescent patient is not immune to reflux sympathetic dystrophy. Therefore, a specific diagnosis is mandatory, and patient expectations of postsurgical results should be discussed preoperatively. The patient with diffuse foot pain is a poor surgical candidate.

Elbow–Radial Head Subluxation

Epidemiology

Subluxation of the head of the radius, also known as "pulled elbow" or "nursemaid's elbow," is subluxation of the annular ligament into the radiohumeral joint. Commonly seen in preschool children 2 to 4 years old, the peak incidence occurs between 1 and 3 years of age. Injury after 5 years of age is rare and is most likely due to abnormal anatomic physiology. Salter and Zaltz[16] found that the annular ligament in children older than 5 years of age is thicker and more firmly attached to the periosteum at the radial neck. Boys are more frequently injured than girls, and the injury is diagnosed more often on the left side than the right side.

Traction may occur when lifting a child by one arm at the wrist or hand or swinging a child by both arms. Although this trauma may be slight, subluxation occurs owing to this longitudinal traction while the elbow is extended and the forearm pronated, resulting in a transverse tear of the annular ligament at its distal attachment to the radial neck. When the forearm is pronated, the radial head has its narrowest diameter in the anteroposterior plane. The radial head protrudes through the tear and migrates distally with proximal recession of the annular ligament into the radiocapitellar joint. Once traction is released, the annular ligament is trapped between the radial head and the capitellum, and full reduction of the radial head is blocked.

Diagnosis

The injured child presents by refusing to use the affected limb but may not complain of pain. Often the shoulder is suspected to be the culprit. At presentation, the arm is held at the side with elbow partially flexed and the forearm pronated. Clinical findings include tenderness to palpation over the radial head and decreased range of motion at the elbow. Radiographs may show soft tissue swelling but are usually negative. Although the elbow is a commonly injured joint in children, interpretation of the radiograph may be difficult owing to joint anatomy. Because the radial epiphysis is not ossified, subluxation is diagnosed on clinical grounds.

Treatment

Reduction of the radial head is possible if the proximal edge of the annular ligament does not extend beyond the widest part of the radial head. Reduction of the annular ligaments is achieved by supination of the forearm, flexion of the elbow, and simultaneous pressure over the radial head. This maneuver is also achieved when manipulating the elbow to obtain an anteroposterior roentgenogram. An audible click may be heard with reduction, associated with significant relief. Often the arm can be used immediately after reduction. Immobility is not necessary. The prognosis is excellent after successful reduction, with only a 5% recurrence rate.[16] On the rare occasion when closed reduction is unsuccessful, surgical referral is warranted. After an open reduction, immobilization of the elbow is recommended in a plaster splint at 90 degrees of flexion with the forearm in neutral position. Mobilization can be started within 1 week.

Classification

The traumatic cause of radial head subluxation, as noted above, is axial traction. In rare cases nontraumatic causes have been identified. Idiopathic subluxation may be due to congenital conditions. In the three cases reported by Southmayd and Ehrlich,[17] the radial head was observed to be enlarged and deformed. Patients presented with no history of trauma but experienced pain and limitation of the range of motion at the elbow. The cause of this condition remains unknown. Other nontraumatic causes of radial head subluxation have been associated with Apert syndrome. In such cases subluxation occurs early, even at birth, and may be the consequence of developmental deformity of abnormal cartilage tissue.

Problems of the Hip and Lower Extremity

Transient Synovitis of the Hip

Transient synovitis of the hip (TSH), a self-limited unilateral disease of unknown etiology, is the most common disorder causing a limp in children. TSH is most common between the ages of 2 and 10 years (average 6 years) and occurs more frequently in boys. The condition often parallels or follows a viral upper respiratory infection and has been considered by some to represent a viral or perhaps "viral-immune response" disorder affecting the hip.[18] The few biopsies reported for this benign, transitory disease have revealed only nonspecific inflammatory congestion and hypertrophy of the synovial membrane.

Children with TSH present with an ill-defined limp, hip or knee pain, and possibly a low-grade fever. The hip is often held flexed, abducted, and externally rotated to provide for maximum joint volume. A complete blood count may show mild leukocytosis without a left shift. The erythrocyte sedimentation rate (ESR) may be elevated, exceeding 20 mm/hour in nearly one third of patients.[19] Radiographs may show capsular swelling characterized by increased distance between the medial acetabulum and the ossified part of the femoral head (Fig. 7.5). Ultrasound examination has been used increasingly as a diagnostic tool to detect hip disorders because of its high sensitivity for demonstrating effusion in the hip joint.

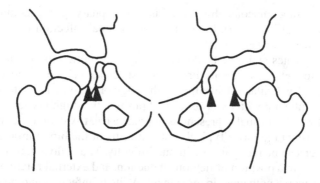

Fig. 7.5. Teardrop distance is the interval between the ossified part of the femoral head or neck and the acetabulum (arrowheads). The teardrop distance is a useful criterion for early diagnosis of Legg–Calvé–Perthes disease and is also a good indicator of the presence of excess joint fluid caused by sepsis. In 96% of normal subjects the teardrop distance in both hips is the same or differs by only 1 mm or less.

It may be difficult to differentiate TSH from early septic arthritis; and if clinical suspicion is high, the hip should be aspirated. Initial treatment is bed rest, usually at home, but occasionally hospitalization is required to perform studies needed to rule out sepsis and thus allay parental and physician concern.

Symptoms may last up to 7 to 10 days but rarely more than 2 weeks. Failure to resolve with rest should lead to a more extensive workup to exclude juvenile rheumatoid arthritis, sacroiliac joint infection, osteomyelitis of the ileum, and osteoid osteoma, each of which may mimic TSH. A few patients with TSH (1–3%) go on to develop Legg–Calvé–Perthes disease within a year.[20] Therefore, patients with TSH should have their hips examined once or twice during the year following acute presentation. Radiographs are unnecessary if hip motion is full.

Septic Hip

A septic hip is considered a medical emergency, as surgical drainage of pus soon after onset of symptoms prevents destruction of the femoral head and neck. Accumulating fluid and pus containing destructive enzymes rapidly elevate the intraarticular pressure and permanently injure vessels and articular cartilage. Microorganisms usually enter the hip joint by bacteremia, the result of distant infection (skin or subcutaneous abscess, otitis media, pharyngitis, pneumonia, or umbilical infection). In neonates nosocomial infection may occur via catheters or venipuncture.

In neonates and infants, the early stages of septic hip may be mistaken for cellulitis, venous thrombosis, superficial abscess, and sciatic nerve palsy. Unilateral swelling of the thigh or leg may indicate a ruptured septic hip with extravasation of pus into the thigh fascial planes. Older children usually present as apprehensive, toxic, and experiencing constant hip pain. Typical septic arthritis of the hip in infants and children can be recognized without difficulty. The child is febrile with the thigh in a position of flexion, abduction, and external rotation. The pain is worse with any hip movement. A site of infection and portal of entry into the bloodstream such as skin abscess, otitis media, or pneumonia is usually present.

Laboratory testing may show an elevated complete blood count (CBC), ESR, and C-reactive protein. C-reactive protein rises within 6 to 8 hours, while the ESR may not rise for 24 to 48 hours. There is considerable overlap between TSH and septic arthritis. No combination of physical exam or laboratory findings is 100% sensitive or specific in diagnosing septic arthritis of the hip.[19] Aspirating pus from the hip joint remains critical for diagnosis and early decompression. Blood cultures and cultures from other sites are obtained before initiating antibiotics (see Reference 51, Chapter 43). *Staphylococcus* and gram-negative organisms are commonly found in newborns. In children 1 to 18 months of age, *Haemophilus influenzae* is a frequent cause of septic hip. *Salmonella* can infect a hip in patients with sickle cell disease. Intravenous antibiotics should be started following needle aspiration and culture, but antibiotics alone cannot cure septic hip. Treatment must include surgical decompression.

Slipped Capital Femoral Epiphysis

Slipped capital femoral epiphysis (SCFE) is the most common serious disorder of the hip in adolescents. The peak age incidence is 11 years for girls and 14 years for boys; the incidence in the general population is approximately 2 per 100,000 with a male to female ratio of 2.5:1.0.[21] SCFE is characterized by sudden or gradual medial displacement of the femoral neck from the capital femoral epiphysis. The epiphysis remains in the acetabulum, resulting in a retroversion deformity of the femoral neck. The goals of treatment for a patient with a SCFE are to stabilize the slip and prevent further displacement while avoiding the complications of avascular necrosis, chondrolysis, and early osteoarthritis.

The etiology is multifactorial and ill-defined. Classification of SCFE has been traditionally based on duration of symptoms. Slips have been divided into acute (symptoms <3 weeks), acute-on-chronic (symptoms of mild pain for >3 weeks with a recent sudden exacerbation), and chronic (symptoms >3 weeks).[22] Newer classification schemes attempt to address the question of stability because unstable slips have a poorer prognosis.[23,24]

With an acute slip, mild symptoms are present for a short time before the displacement occurs; minimal trauma may then cause an acute separation, with pain so severe the child cannot bear weight on the affected side. Patients with the chronic form have hip pain localized to the groin, buttock, or lateral hip. Occasionally, the child has only knee pain. There is a decrease in abduction, flexion, and internal rotation, and as the hip is gently flexed it may roll into external rotation.

The clinical diagnosis of SCFE requires radiographic confirmation of femoral head displacement. Radiographic assessment must include both hips in anteroposterior (AP) and lateral views. Both hips are included because bilateral disease occurs in one third of cases.[25] The earliest changes may be subtle, only showing widening or irregularity of the epiphyseal plate (Fig. 7.6). Since initial displacement occurs posteriorly, the true lateral or "frog" lateral views are most sensitive to detect early SCFE. On the AP view the Klein's line drawn along the superior femoral neck should intersect 20% of the lateral femoral head (Fig. 7.6). When the diagnosis is suspected from the clinical findings, but plain radiographs are not conclusive, magnetic resonance imaging (MRI) is the best study to demonstrate the subtle widening and irregularity of the physis and even early slippage of the femoral head.[26]

Surgery is the only reliable treatment for SCFE. Results are best if it is performed soon after diagnosis because outcomes depend on early stabilization. Any attempt to reduce a chronic slip produces avascular necrosis.

In children who have unilateral disease at diagnosis, nearly 20% may go on to develop bilateral disease. Most often sequential slips will occur within 18 months, although reports have documented cases that occur up to 5 years after initial diagnosis.[25] Frequent follow-up examination is recommended until definite radiographic evidence of physeal closure is noted.

Developmental Dysplasia of the Hip

The term *developmental dysplasia of the hip* (DDH) describes a spectrum of disorders: frank dislocation, partial dislocation (subluxation),

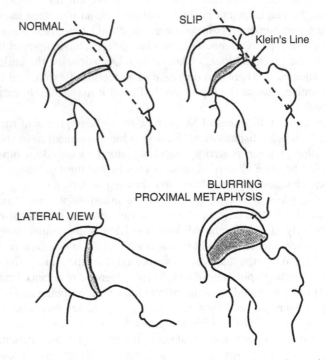

Fig. 7.6. Left slipped capital femoral epiphysis. A line drawn along the superior aspect of the femoral neck (Klein's line) barely intersects with the femoral head compared to the normal right side, a sign of slipping of the left femoral head.

instability, and acetabular dysplasia. Because many of these findings are not present at birth, the term *developmental dysplasia* has replaced the older term *congenital hip dislocation*. The reported incidence of all forms of DDH is 2 to 6/1000 and is influenced by genetic and environmental factors. The etiology of DDH is multifactorial. The female to male ratio is 5:1. Hormonal factors play a role in joint laxity. Mechanical factors increasing the risk of DDH include oligohydramnios, primigravida, and breech presentation. Intrauterine positioning may explain the 3:1 predominance of left hip involvement. One in five children with DDH has a positive family history.[27,28]

In the newborn, Barlow and Ortolani tests (Fig. 7.7) are the most reliable tests for diagnosis and should be part of every well-baby examination (see Reference 51, Chapter 17). The infant is examined relaxed and supine, with one of the examiner's hands stabilizing the pelvis. The other hand holds the hip to be examined with the thumb in the groin and the index or long finger over the greater trochanter. The hip is flexed to 90 degrees and adducted past the midline while a gentle outward force is made by the thumb. The hip may be felt to dislocate during adduction (positive Barlow sign). The hip is then abducted and gently lifted. Relocation of the dislocated femoral head may be felt (a pop is not heard), which is a positive Ortolani's

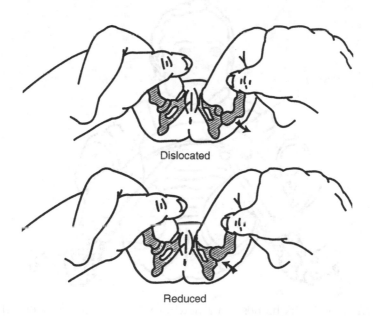

Dislocated

Reduced

Fig. 7.7. Barlow and Ortolani tests.

reduction test. A positive test is felt as a "clunk." The high-pitched click that is often heard is normal and unrelated to DDH.

In the child over 2 to 3 months of age, muscle tightness may mask dislocation or reduction. Clinical signs are more subtle as the child approaches walking age, but the following abnormalities should always be sought during well-child examinations: an asymmetric hip abduction, one knee lower than the other (positive Galeazzi's sign), and asymmetric thigh creases. Unfortunately, these clinical examinations do not identify all neonates with DDH, in part because some cases are missed on initial examination and other children develop instability later. Standard radiographs are difficult to interpret until the femoral head begins to ossify at 3 to 6 months of age. During dynamic ultrasonography a modified Barlow maneuver is used for the hip evaluation, increasing the accuracy of diagnosing hip instability after 6 weeks of age.[29,30]

Neonatal hip instability or dislocation can be treated with a Pavlik-type harness (Fig. 7.8) with 85% to 90% success in infants up to 6 to 8 months of age.[31,32] This harness holds the infant's hips in a flexed and abducted position, directing the femoral head into the developing acetabulum. Pavlik harness use requires close ultrasound or radiographic monitoring and frequent clinical follow-up. Most hips stabi-

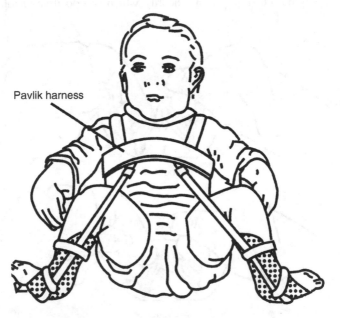

Pavlik harness

Fig. 7.8. Pavlik harness on a newborn. The hips are fully flexed, then fall out passively into abduction.

lize after 2 to 3 months. Dislocated hips diagnosed at 6 to 18 months of age often require closed or open surgical reduction under anesthesia, followed by spica cast immobilization.

Legg–Calvé–Perthes Disease

Legg–Calvé–Perthes disease (LCPD) is avascular necrosis of the femoral head in otherwise clinically normal children. LCPD typically presents between 4 and 8 years of age, with the boy/girl ratio approximately 5:1. Bilateral involvement occurs in approximately 10%.[20] Interesting parallels exist between LCPD and "constitutional delay of growth." Children with LCPD are often small for age, and thin, with bone age that is delayed by 1 to 2 years. Recent studies have proposed a link with familial thrombotic disorders, such as the factor V Leiden mutation.[33] Age at onset is an important indicator of outcome; children under 6 years of age often do well without specific treatment, whereas children over 9 years have a worse prognosis.[20]

Catterall[34] has classified LCPD according to radiographic findings of the percent of the femoral head that is avascular. The ultimate Catterall classification may not be determined for 6 to 9 months after the initial onset.[35] The history and physical findings can vary markedly depending on the stage of the disease process. During the early stages, the history is most often that of a limp or increasing groin, thigh, or knee pain. The physical findings at this time are similar to those of a child with an "irritable hip"; the initial synovitis may cause a decrease in range of motion on internal and external rotation, and there may be muscle atrophy of the thigh or calf consistent with an antalgic gait. With later, more severe stages of LCPD, there may be contractures of the adductor and hip flexor musculature in addition to restricted internal and external rotation.

Techniques for diagnosing LCPD and determining its prognosis include radiography, technetium scanning, MRI, arthrography, and CT scans. They are all equally useful, and each has advantages and disadvantages. Laboratory evaluation is normal.

LCPD is a self-healing disorder and there is no evidence that any treatment speeds the return of blood flow to the femoral head.[20] The main treatment objectives are to relieve muscle spasm, regain range of motion, and contain the femoral epiphysis within the acetabulum to minimize deformation of the femoral head. Orthopedic consultation is recommended. Nonsurgical treatment includes the use of a spica cast, removable orthosis, and braces. Surgical options for more severe disease include soft tissue procedures to release the adductors and bony procedures to mechanically realign the hip.[36] Long-term outcomes are good for most children, although approximately 10% to 15% develop deteriorating symptoms and degenerative arthritis that may require hip arthroplasty.[37] Most patients with LCPD can participate in sports.

Apophyseal Injuries

Apophysitis of the Hip

Apophyseal injury involving the anterosuperior and anteroinferior iliac spines, iliac crest, and ischial tuberosity typically occurs in active adolescents. Major abdominal and hip muscles either insert or originate at these sites of bone growth. The condition is most common in distance runners and dancers and is associated with muscle–tendon imbalance and rapid growth (see Chapter 10). Adolescents present with vague, dull pain related to activity located near the hip. Should a single traumatic episode exceed the strength of the physis, an avulsion fracture through the growth plate occurs. Radiographs may be useful for evaluating acute trauma and ruling out other hip pathology. Treatment includes rest from the offending activity followed by a program of stretching and progressive strengthening of the abdominal and hip muscles (Table 7.1). Depending on their size and displacement, acute fractures may be treated with rest or open-reduction internal fixation.

Sinding–Larsen–Johansson Syndrome

Sinding–Larsen–Johansson syndrome is an apophyseal injury to the inferior pole of the patella. The condition is thought to result from multiple episodes of traction-induced microtrauma at an immature, inferior patellar pole, with resultant calcification and ossification at this junction. It is commonly seen in active preteen boys (10–12 years old), who complain of pain over the inferior pole of the patella or at the proximal quadriceps patellar junction that is worsened by running or stair climbing. Point tenderness is noted at the patella–quadriceps or patella–patellar tendon junctions. The remainder of the knee examination is usually normal. Radiographs may be normal or show varying amounts and shapes of calcification or ossification at the patellar junction.

It is important to advise the patient and family that it is a self-limited condition that improves with rest and attainment of skeletal maturity. Activity modification, use of a knee sleeve, ice, massage, and antiinflammatory medication are usually helpful for reducing discomfort.

Table 7.1. **Apophyseal Injuries**

Injury	Age (years)	Site	Presentation	Differential diagnosis	Treatment
Sever's disease	8–13	Posterior calcaneus	Heel pain with activity	Achilles tendinitis, stress fracture	Heel cups, RICE, decrease activity, NSAIDs
Osgood–Schlatter disease	Boys: 10–15 Girls: 8–13	Tibial tuberosity	Anterior knee pain	PFD, OCD, stress fracture	RICE, activity modification, NSAIDs
Sindig–Larsen–Johannson syndrome	10–13	Inferior pole of patella	Anterior knee pain	PFD, OCD, stress fracture	RICE, activity modification NSAIDs
Apophysitis of the hip	9–13	ASIS, AIIS, iliac crest, ischial tuberosity	Dull ache around the hip	Muscle strain, stress fracture	RICE, stretching program, NSAIDs

Source: Peck,[53] with permission.

NSAIDs = nonsteroidal antiinflammatory drugs; PFD = patellofemoral dysfunction; OCD = osteochondritis dissecans; RICE = rest, ice, compression, and elevation; ASIS = anterosuperior iliac spine; AIIS = anteroinferior iliac spine.

Osgood–Schlatter Disease

Osgood–Schlatter disease, the most common apophyseal disorder, was independently described in 1903.[38] The condition is found most commonly in boys age 10 to 15 years and in girls 2 years earlier; it is often bilateral (20–30% of cases). On examination, exquisite tenderness may be noted over the anterior tibial tubercle, with prominence and swelling at that location. Pain worsens during running, jumping, and ascending or descending stairs. Resisted extension of the knee at 90 degrees of flexion causes pain. Radiographs are obtained to exclude the possibility of osteomyelitis and arterial-venous malformations. A discrete separate ossicle is noted at the tibial tubercle in as many as 50% of reported cases.

The patient and family must understand that 12 to 18 months may be required to allow spontaneous resolution by physiologic epiphysiodesis. Treatment with ice, antiinflammatory medication, and an appropriately contoured knee pad relieves symptoms. The level of sporting activity is balanced with tolerance and severity of symptoms. If symptoms progress to disability with activities of daily living, a brief course (7–10 days) of knee immobilization usually resolves the discomfort. Steroid injections into the tibial tubercle should never be done. Rare, persistent cases that fail to respond to a lengthy trial of conservative therapy may resolve with surgical removal of the bony ossicle overlying the tibial tubercle.

Sever's Disease

In 1912 Sever[39] described a benign inflammatory condition to the calcaneal apophysis in active adolescents. The sports most commonly associated with Sever's disease are soccer and running. The disease presents with unilateral or bilateral (60%) posterior heel pain in the 8- to 13-year-old athlete. It is associated with accelerated growth, tight heel cords, and other biomechanical abnormalities. Patients present with tenderness at the insertion of the Achilles tendon on the calcaneus. Radiographs may show partial fragmentation and increased density of the os calcis, thereby ruling out other rare causes of heel pain, such as unicameral bone cyst or a stress fracture. Activity modification, stretching of the gastrocnemius–soleus complex, ankle inverters and everters, and heel cups have all proved helpful. Children may return to sports without limitation 2 to 4 weeks after symptoms resolve.

Osteochondritis Dissecans

Osteochondritis dissecans (OCD) is characterized by separation of a fragment of bone with overlying articular cartilage from the surrounding normal bone. OCD most commonly affects the medial aspect of the lateral femoral condyle, but is also seen in the talar dome and humeral capitellum (Fig 7.9). OCD can occur in all large joints. The incidence is estimated to be 15 to 30 cases per 100,000 persons. OCD may be more common than is currently known because asymptomatic lesions are discovered only incidentally. Risk factors include repetitive microtrauma as seen in throwing sports or gymnastics. OCD has a familial predisposition. Contralateral joint involvement is noted in 20% to 30% of patients with OCD of the knee.

Without proper management the disease may progress through four stages: stage 1, thickening of the articular cartilage (stable); stage 2, fragment in situ and beginning of demarcation of the articular cartilage (stable); stage 3, partial detachment (unstable); and stage 4, complete detachment of the fragment and formation of a loose body (unstable).[40] OCD may be viewed as a stress fracture of the involved subchondral bone and requires differentiation from epiphyseal dysplasia, ossification defects, and acute osteochondral fracture. Symptoms include vague joint pain, catching, restricted range of motion, and pain with activity or range of motion. Plain radiographs reveal most lesions. Radioisotope scanning may be used if onset is acute and x rays are negative. MRI is the gold standard for staging once the diagnosis is made.

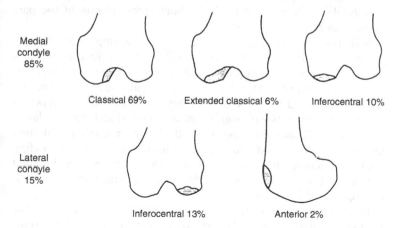

Fig. 7.9. Distribution of osteochondritis dissecans by body location.

Conservative treatment, including avoidance of stressful or painful activities and restricted weight bearing for periods ranging from 2 to 6 months may be successful in selected patients. Predictors of good clinical outcomes with conservative management include open joint physis, and small lesions that are stable on MRI.[41] Not all lesions heal spontaneously, and surgery may be required to stimulate new bone growth. Most orthopedic surgeons prefer arthroscopic drilling of the lesion from inside the joint.

Problems of the Spine

Spondylolysis and Spondylolisthesis

Spondylolysis is an acquired condition in which there is a bony defect on one or both sides of the pars interarticularis (Fig. 7.10), usually at the L5-S1 level. The incidence of spondylolysis is about 5% in preadolescent North American children and rises to 12% in gymnasts and divers.[42] The defect is not apparent at birth but develops usually between 5 and 10 years of age.[43] Thus vigorous athletic activity in children may produce repetitive stress on the developing pars. When bilateral pars defects are present at a single vertebral level, translation (slip) of the vertebral body may occur in adjacent vertebrae, which is termed spondylolisthesis. Four distinct types of spondylolisthesis have been described: dysplastic, isthmic, degenerative, and traumatic. Most cases in children and adolescents are of the dysplastic or isthmic type, whereas degenerative changes of the facet joints may result in spondylolisthesis in older adults without spondylolysis of the pars interarticularis.

Spondylolysis and spondylolisthesis may be asymptomatic or may present with low back pain occasionally radiating to the buttocks. Physical examination may show lumbosacral tenderness and accentuation of pain by hyperextension of the spine with one leg raised off the ground and flexed 90 degrees at the hip and knee (one-leg hyperextension test). Patients with significant spondylolisthesis have a classic appearance of a short torso and flat buttocks, often standing with their knees held in modest extension. Neurological status, including bladder function, must be assessed, although neurological deficit is unusual and is seen in about 35% of those with more than 50% slippage of the vertebrae.[43]

Radiographs should include anteroposterior, lateral, and oblique views of the lumbar spine. The pars defect is best seen on the oblique film (Fig. 7.10) and is unilateral in about 20% of patients. The pars defect appears as a band or break in the "Scotty dog's neck" (pars

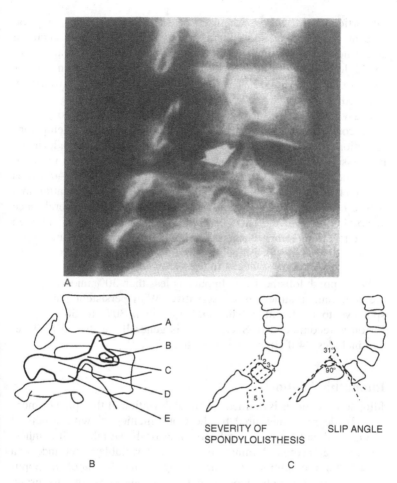

Fig. 7.10. Spondylolysis, and spondylolisthesis (right). (A) Radiographic representation of an abnormal elongation (greyhound sign) of the pars interarticularis, or the "neck" of a scotty dog (arrow). Other defects, such as sclerosis or lysis in the pars, are best visualized in this "neck." (From Lillegard and Kruse,[50] with permission.) (B) "Scotty dog." A = superior articular process (ear); B = pedicle (eye); C = pars interarticularis (neck); D = lamina (body); E = inferior articular process (front leg). (C) Severity of spondylolisthesis and slip angle.

interarticularis) of L5. Sclerosis of the opposite pars may be present. A standing spot lateral view of L5-S1 allows accurate assessment of a possible slip. Scoliosis is commonly associated with spondylolisthesis. Bone scans show increased activity on one or both sides in symptomatic spondylolysis but are not routinely required.

If asymptomatic, no treatment is required, and there is no need to limit contact sports. For a mildly symptomatic patient, temporary reduction of activity is all that is needed. If symptoms are alleviated, progressive activity is permitted. Symptoms that are sudden in onset, traumatically induced, or do not resolve with rest do heal—much as any fracture would heal—after 10 to 12 weeks of immobilization in a plastic body jacket or a Boston-type spinal orthosis. In general, once symptoms resolve, the child can resume normal activities, although advice regarding return to rigorous spine-bending athletic events (gymnastics, diving, downed lineman in football) is controversial (see Chapter 10).

With spondylolisthesis, if slippage is less than 30% and symptoms are minimal, treatment is conservative. With persistent pain unresponsive to treatment or slippage more than 30% to 50%, spinal fusion is recommended. Such fusion is generally at the L5-S1 level and includes L4 if slippage is more than 50%.[44]

Idiopathic Scoliosis

Idiopathic scoliosis is defined as lateral deviation of the spine of more than 10 degrees (measured by the Cobb method),[45] with structural change and without congenital anomalies of the vertebrae. It is inherited in an autosomal-dominant manner with variable penetrance or a multifactorial condition. It occurs in approximately 2% of the population. Normally, only about one fifth to one sixth of this group require treatment.[46]

Scoliosis is a painless condition usually identified by shoulder, scapular, or pelvic asymmetry during school screening or routine physical examination. Forward bending (Adam's) testing is done with the child standing straight and bending forward with palms together and knees straight. Truncal asymmetry, most commonly right rib prominence, may be seen. Any limb length irregularity should be noted and corrected by placing blocks under the short leg and leveling the pelvis prior to examination. Neurological examination is normal. Initial radiological evaluation consists of standing PA and lateral spine films on a long cassette to include the pelvis. The curve is measured using the Cobb method[45] (Fig. 7.11). If a structural curve of 10

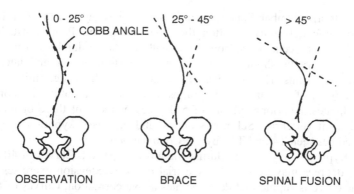

Fig. 7.11. Measuring the Cobb angle and treatment of idiopathic scoliosis.

to 20 degrees is identified, orthopedic referral is recommended. Painful scoliosis or an atypical curve pattern (apex left thoracic) is indicative of possible underlying neurological problems, such as syringomyelia or spinal cord lesion, and is probably not idiopathic scoliosis.

The risk of curve progression is higher in young children, in those with large curves or double curves, and in girls. Bracing is usually initiated for curves of more than 20 degrees with documented progression and growth remaining or for curves initially 30 degrees or more. Curves of more than 45 to 50 degrees are usually not amenable to bracing, so surgery is recommended, as the risk of continued progression after skeletal maturity is high in this group.[46]

Scheuermann's Disease

Scheuermann's disease (juvenile kyphosis) is defined as an abnormal increase in thoracic kyphosis (normal 20–40 degrees) during puberty with at least 5 degrees of anterior wedging of at least three or more adjacent vertebrae. It is to be distinguished from postural round back, which is more flexible and lacks radiographical changes in the vertebrae.[47] The etiology is unclear, but a familial incidence is noted in 30% to 48% of cases. It occurs in about 1% of the population and is more common in boys.

Clinically, it is possible to distinguish two forms of juvenile kyphosis. Thoracic Scheuermann's disease has an apex of the curve at T7–9, and thoracolumbar Scheuermann's disease has an apex at T11-12. Cosmetic deformity is often the chief complaint. Pain is usually aching and occurs more commonly with the thoracolumbar form.

Radiographs should include standing posteroanterior and lateral scoliosis films. Hyperextension lateral films help to determine the flexibility of the curve. Radiographs show irregularity of the vertebral endplates, anterior wedging of 5 degrees or more of three or more adjacent vertebrae, Schmorl's nodes, and increased kyphosis measured between T4 and T12 by the Cobb method.

Kyphosis may worsen during the growing period. Curves of 40 to 60 degrees may be treated by a trial of hyperextension exercises if the curve is supple and demonstrates active correction. Curves of 60 to 75 degrees are treated with a Milwaukee brace or underarm orthosis with a breastplate. Bracing is begun if the vertebral end plates are not fused to the vertebral body, with full-time wearing for 6 to 12 months and then part-time (about 16 hours/day) for 6 months or until the end plate fuses. Bracing is less effective for curves of more than 65 to 75 degrees or after skeletal maturity. Surgery may be indicated for cosmesis, progressive deformity despite bracing, or intractable pain. No long-term cardiopulmonary problems have been identified.[48,49]

References

1. Karoll LA. Rotational deformities in the lower extremities. Curr Opin Pediatr 1997;9:77–90.
2. Engel FM, Staheli LT. The natural history of torsion and other factors influencing gait in early childhood. Clin Orthop 1974;99: 12–17.
3. Wells L. Common lower extremity problems in children, primary care. Clin Office Pract 1996;23(2):299–303.
4. Brink DS, Levitsky DR. Cuneiform and cuboid wedge osteotomies for correction of residual metatarsus adductus: a surgical review. J Foot Ankle Surg 1995;34:371–8.
5. Fabray G, MacEwen GD, Shands AR Jr. Torsion of the femur: a follow-up study in normal and abnormal conditions. J Bone Joint Surg 1973;55A:1726–38.
6. Kling TF, Hensinger RN. Angular and torsional deformities of the lower limbs in children. Clin Orthop 1983;176:136–47.
7. Bruce RW Jr. Torsional and angular deformities. Pediatr Clin North Am 1996;43(4):867–81.
8. Mielke CH, Stevens PM. Hemiepiphyseal stapling for knee deformities in children younger than 10 years: a preliminary report. J Pediatr Orthop 1996;16:423–9.

9. Cummings RJ, Lovell WW. Operative treatment of congenital idiopathic club foot. J Bone Joint Surg 1988;70A:1108–12.

10. Ponseti IV. Congenital clubfoot, the results of treatment. J Bone Joint Surg 1963;45A:261–9.

11. Cowell H. Talocalcaneal coalition and new causes of peroneal spastic flatfoot. Clin Orthop 1972;85:16–22.

12. Hoffinger SA. Evaluation and management of pediatric foot deformities. Pediatr Clin North Am 1996;43:1091–111.

13. Paulos L, Samuelson KM. Pes cavovarus: review of a surgical approach using selective soft tissue procedures. J Bone Joint Surg 1980;62A:942–53.

14. Wenger DR, Mauldin D, Speck G, Morgan D, Lieber R. Corrective shoes and inserts as treatment for flexible flatfoot in infants and children. J Bone Joint Surg 1989;71A:800–10.

15. Steward M. Miscellaneous afflictions of the foot. In: Campbell's operative orthopedics. St. Louis: Mosby, 1980;1703.

16. Salter RB, Zaltz C. Anatomic investigation of the mechanism of injury and pathologic anatomy of "pulled elbow" in young children. Clin Orthop 1971;77:134.

17. Southmayd W, Ehrlich MB. Idiopathic subluxation of the radial head. Clin Orthop 1976;121:271.

18. Hardinse K. The etiology of transient synovitis of the hip in childhood. J Bone Joint Surg 1970;52B:100–7.

19. Del Beccaro M, Champoux A, Bockers T, Mendelman P. Septic arthritis versus transient synovitis of the hip: The value of screening laboratory tests. Ann Emerg Med 1992;21(12):1418–22.

20. Roy DR. Current concepts in Legg-Calve-Perthes Disease. Pediatr Ann 1999;28(12):748–52.

21. Busch M, Morrisy R. Slipped capital femoral epiphysis. Orthop Clin North Am 1987;18:637–47.

22. Fahey JJ, O'Brien ET. Acute slipped capital femoral epiphysis: review of the literature and report of ten cases. J Bone Joint Surg 1965;47A: 1105–27.

23. Kallio PE, Paterson DC, Foster BK, Lequene GW. Classification in slipped capital femoral epiphysis. Clin Orthop 1993;294:196–203.

24. Loder RT, Richards BS, Shapiro PS, Reznick LR, Aronsson DD. Acute slipped capital femoral epiphysis: the importance of physical stability. J Bone Joint Surg 1993;75A:1134–40.

25. Loder RT, Aronson DD, Greenfield ML. The epidemiology of bilateral slipped capital femoral epiphysis. J Bone Joint Surg 1993;75A:1141–7.

26. Umas H, Liebling M, Moy L, Harmamati N, Macy N, Pritzker H. Slipped capital femoral epiphysis: a physeal lesion diagnosed by MRI, with radiographic and CT correlation. Skel Radiol 1998;27.139–44.

27. Committee on Quality Improvement and Subcommittee on Developmental Dysplasia of the Hip. American Academy of Pediatrics: clinical practice guideline: early detection of developmental dysplasia of the hip. Pediatrics 2000;105(4):896–905.

28. Gerscovich EO. Radiologists' guide to the imaging in the diagnosis and treatment of developmental dysplasia of the hip. Skel Radiol 1997; 26:386–97.

29. Rosendahl K, Markestad T, Lie RT. Ultrasound in the early diagnosis of congenital dislocation of the hip: the significance of hip stability versus acetabular morphology. Pediatr Radiol 1992;22:430–3.

30. Graf R. Hip semiography: how reliable? Sector scanning versus linear scanning? Dynamic versus static examination? Clin Orthop 1992;281: 18–21.

31. Weinstein SL. Congenital hip dislocation: long-range problems, residual signs and symptoms after successful treatment. Clin Orthop 1992; 281:69–74.

32. Harris IE, Dickens R, Menelaus MB. Use of the Pavlic harness for hip displacements: when to abandon treatment. Clin Orthop 1992; 281:29–33.

33. Gruppo R, Glueck CJ, Wall E, Roy D, Wang P. Legg-Perthes disease in three siblings, two heterozygous and one homozygous for the factor V Leiden mutation. J Pediatr 1998;132(5):885–8.

34. Catterall A. The natural history of Perthes' disease. J Bone Joint Surg 1971;53B:37–53.

35. Gershuni DH. Preliminary evaluation and prognosis in Legg-Calvé-Perthes disease. Clin Orthop 1980;150:16–22.

36. Herring JA. The treatment of Legg-Calve-Perthes disease. J Bone Joint Surg 1994;76A(3):448–57.

37. McAndrew MP. Weinstein SL. A long-term follow-up of Legg-Calve-Perthes disease. J Bone Joint Surg 1984;66A(6):860–9.

38. Osgood RB. Lesions of the tibial tubercle occurring during adolescence. Boston Med J 1903;148:114–17.

39. Sever JW. Apophysitis of the os calcis. NY Med J 1912;95: 1025–9.

40. Obedian RS, Grelsamer RP. Osteochondritis dissecans of the distal femur and patella. Clin Sports Med 1997;16:157–74.

41. De Smet AA. Omer AI, Graf BK. Untreated osteochondritis dissecans of the femoral condyles: prediction of patient outcome using radiographic and MR findings. Skel Radiol 1997;26:463–7.

42. Wiltse LL, Newman PH, Macnab I. Classification of spondylolysis and spondylolisthesis. Clin Orthop 1976;117:23–9.

43. Hensinger RN. Spondylolysis and spondylolisthesis in children and adolescents. J Bone Joint Surg 1989;71A:1098–107.

44. Boxall D, Bradford DS, Winter RB, Moe JH. Management of severe spondylolisthesis in children and adolescents. J Bone Joint Surg 1979;61:479–95.

45. Sorensen KH. Scheuermann's juvenile kyphosis. Copenhagen: Munksgaard, 1964.

46. Hensinger RN, Greene TL, Hunter LY. Back pain and vertebral changes simulating Scheuermann's kyphosis. Spine 1982;6:341–2.

47. Bradford DS. Juvenile kyphosis. In: Bradford DS, Lonstein JE, Moe JH, et al, eds. Moe's textbook of scoliosis and other spinal deformities, 2nd ed. Philadelphia: WB Saunders, 1987;347–68.

48. Cobb J. Outline for study of scoliosis. AAOS Instruct Course Lect 1948;5:261–275, Ann Arbor: J. W. Edwards.

49. Moe JH, Byrd JA III. Idiopathic scoliosis. In: Bradford DS, Lonstein JH, Moe JH, et al, eds. Moe's textbook of scoliosis and other spinal deformities, 2nd ed. Philadelphia: WB Saunders, 1987;191–232.
50. Lillegard W, Kruse R. In Taylor RB, eds. Family medicine: principles and practice, 4th ed. New York: Springer-Verlag, 1993.
51. Taylor RB. Family medicine: principles and practice, 6th ed. New York: Springer-Verlag, 2003.
52. Gerberg LF, Micheli LJ, Nontraumatic hip pain in active children: a critical differential. Phys Sports Med 1996;24:69–74.
53. Peck DM. Apophyseal injuries in the young athlete. Am Fam phys 1995;51:1891–5.

8
Osteoporosis

Paula Cifuentes Henderson and Richard P. Usatine

Osteoporosis is a major health concern affecting approximately 20 million people in the United States. It is responsible for more than 1.3 million fractures annually,[1] with $15 billion in direct financial expenditures to treat these fractures.[2] The clinical consequences of an osteoporotic fracture include increased mortality, disability, and the need for long-term nursing care. After a hip fracture the mortality rate of patients 65 to 79 years old at 1 year is between 20% and 30%, and these rates worsen with increased age.[3] Among those who survive, 50% won't be able to work without some type of assistance. After a collapsed osteoporotic vertebra, 30% of patients will experience chronic disabling back pain and spinal deformity.[4,5] Osteoporotic fractures have a profound impact on quality of life, decreasing the physical, functional, and psychological performance secondary to pain, deformities, and inability to perform the activities of daily living (ADL)[6].

Osteoporosis is a disease characterized by low bone mass and microarchitectural deterioration of bone tissue leading to enhanced bone fragility and a consequent increase in fracture risk.[7] It can be a silent disease because it is often asymptomatic until a fracture occurs. The lifetime risk of a 50-year-old white woman of having an osteoporotic fracture is 40%. Fractures secondary to osteoporosis are more common in women than in men and in Caucasians and Asians than in African Americans and Latinos.[8] These fractures most commonly occur at the hip, vertebrae, and wrists.

Primary osteoporosis is related to aging and not associated with chronic illness. Secondary osteoporosis is related to chronic conditions that contribute to accelerated bone loss such as with hyperparathyroidism, malignancy, renal failure, and hyperthyroidism.[9]

Assessment and Diagnosis

Risk Factor Assessment

Start with the medical history and ask questions about:

Menopause (surgical and natural)
Family history of osteoporosis (especially mother)
Exercise
Diet
Smoking
Alcohol intake

Other risk factors such as age, gender, ethnicity, and slender body habitus can usually be observed without asking specific questions. The physical exam includes the measurement of height and weight, and the examination of the spine looking for any signs of deformity such as kyphosis, scoliosis, and limited range of motion. Screening for secondary forms of osteoporosis may be helpful. Assess the patient's risk of falling by asking about a history of falls and a decrease in visual acuity.[10,11]

Genetic Issues

The prevalence of osteoporosis varies by sex, ethnicity, and race.[12] Decreased bone density is more common in women of Northern European or Asian descent. Women and men experience age-related decrease in bone mass density starting at midlife, but women experience more rapid bone loss after the menopause.[13] Genetic syndromes like Turner's (45,X0) syndrome patients have streak ovaries and decreased estrogen production leading to the early development of osteoporosis.[14]

Endocrine Factors

Risk factors associated with decreased bone density include early estrogen deficiency secondary to surgery or to early menopause, hyperthyroidism, hyperparathyroidism, hypercortisolism, Addison's disease, and Cushing's syndrome.[14]

Medications

Chronic use of certain medications that affect the bone metabolism, such as corticosteroids, exogenous thyroid hormone, gonadotropin-releasing hormone (GnRH) analogues, anticoagulants, and anticonvulsants, increase the risk of osteoporosis and subsequent fractures.[15]

Lifestyle

Excessive use of alcohol depresses osteoblastic function and increases the risk of osteoporosis. Physical activity early in life contributes to higher peak bone mass and reduces the risk of falls by approximately 25%.[16] Good nutrition with a balanced diet is necessary for the development of healthy bones. Calcium and vitamin D are required for the prevention and treatment of osteoporosis. There are data to support recommendations (found later in the chapter) for specific dietary calcium intakes at various stages in life.[17,18] Patients at high risk also include those who pursue thinness excessively, have a history of an eating disorder,[19] restrict their intake of dairy products, don't consume enough vegetables and fruits, and have a high intake of low-calcium/high-phosphorus beverages like sodas. These beverages have a negative effect on calcium balance.

Laboratory Assessment

If the history and physical exam suggests secondary causes of osteoporosis, the physician should consider tests such as thyroid-stimulating hormone (TSH), parathyroid hormone (PTH), calcium, vitamin D, urine N-teloptide, complete blood count (CBC), chem panel, cortisol, erythrocyte sedimentation rate (ESR), or serum protein electrophoresis, based on the differential diagnosis.[20,21]

Bone Densitometry Assessment

To prevent osteoporosis, the physician should attempt to establish early detection of low bone mineral density (BMD). Currently there is no accurate measure of bone strength, but BMD is the accepted method to establish a diagnosis of osteoporosis and predict future fracture risk.[22,23] The World Health Organization (WHO) defines osteoporosis as a BMD 2.5 standard deviations (SDs) below the mean for young white adult women. This definition does not apply to other ethnic groups, men, or children.[7,24] The U.S. Preventive Services Task Force suggests that the primary reason to screen postmenopausal women is to check for a low BMD so that early intervention may be initiated to slow the further decrease of the bone density.[25] The ultimate goal is to prevent vertebral and hip fractures.

The most thoroughly studied and most widely used technique to measure BMD is the dual-energy x-ray absortiometry (DEXA) scan. This is considered to be the gold standard screening test to measure the BMD of the hip and spine. It is less expensive and involves less radiation exposure than the quantitative computed tomography (CT). Since some patients don't respond to therapy for osteoporosis, the BMD results can also be used to follow them and evaluate their response to treatment. Bone mass should be measured in postmenopausal women 1 to 2 years following the initiation of therapy.

The report of the DEXA provides a T score and a Z score. The T score is defined as the number of SDs above or below the mean BMD for sex- and race-matched young controls (not age matched). This should be distinguished from a Z score, which is defined as the number of SDs above or below the average BMD comparing the patient with the population adjusted for age, sex, and race. These results can be used to classify patients into three categories: normal, osteopenic, and osteoporotic (Table 8.1). Osteoporosis is diagnosed using the patient's T score, because the T score is a measure of current fracture risk. A T score of 1 SD below the age-predicted mean is associated with a two- to threefold increased risk of fracture. Patients with T scores more than 2 SDs below the mean have an exponential increase in their risk of fracture. Z scores have little significant value for clinical practice.

Newer measures of bone strength, such as the ultrasound, are being introduced as an alternative screening method to the DEXA scan. This measurement of bone mass is being done through peripheral bone mass assessment. In 1998, the Food and Drug Administration (FDA) approved the use of a portable ultrasound to

Table 8.1. **World Health Organization (WHO) Diagnostic Criteria for Osteoporosis**

Diagnosis	Bone Mineral Density (BMD) T score[a]
Normal	≤1
Osteopenia	1–2.5
Osteoporosis	≥2.5
Severe osteoporosis	≥2.5 and history of fracture

[a]Standard deviation (SD) below the mean in healthy young adults.
Source: WHO Study Group.[7]

assess bone mass through the measurement of the calcaneous. If a patient has a low T score in the ultrasound of a peripheral bone, the current recommendation is to obtain a DEXA of the hip and spine for further evaluation and treatment.[11]

The diagnosis and treatment of osteoporosis should be individualized based on each patient's risk factors rather than the assessment of a T score alone.

Indications for bone mineral density assessment include:

Women ≥65 years old who are willing to start drug therapy if BMD is found to be low

Women <65 who have at least one additional risk factor for osteoporosis

Postmenopausal women with a fracture

Radiographic evidence of bone loss

Long-term steroid use

Hyperparathyroidism

Monitoring therapeutic response if the results would affect the clinical decision.

Although there is no evidence to support this, some clinicians screen premenopausal women with BMD for the following conditions:

Prolonged oligo/amenorrhea

A long-standing history of eating disorders

Stress fractures

Chronic use of medications that promote bone resorption.

There is a lack of evidence to support the cost-effectiveness of universal routine bone density screenings or to support the efficacy of early preventive medications to prevent fractures. Therefore, an individualized approach is recommended[25] (Table 8.2).

Bone Remodeling Assessment

Another way to assess bone strength is to measure markers of bone remodeling (turnover) in the blood or urine. There is some evidence that bone turnover rate predicts the risk of osteoporotic fractures in postmenopausal women.[26] These markers include indices of bone resorption such as serum and urine levels of C- and N-telopeptide, and indices of bone formation such as osteocalcin and bone-specific alkaline phosphatase. These markers of bone turnover may be particularly

Table 8.2. **Indications for Bone Mineral Density (BMD) Screening**

National Osteoporosis Foundation guidelines[a]
   Women >65 willing to start therapy if BMD low
   Women <65 postmenopausal with at least one additional risk factor
   All postmenopausal women with fractures
   Women considering therapy for osteoporosis, and BMD would affect
      decision
   Women who have received HRT for a prolonged period
   No formal guideline developed in premenopausal women

American Association of Clinical Endocrinologists clinical practice
      guidelines[b]
   Perimenopausal women willing to start therapy if BMD low
   X-ray evidence of bone loss
   Asymptomatic hyperparathyroidism
   Monitoring therapeutic response and BMD would affect decision
   Long-term use of glucocorticoid

BMD = bone mineral density; HRT = hormone replacement therapy.

[a]National Osteoporosis Foundation (NOF). Physician's guide to prevention and treatment of osteoporosis. Washington, DC: NOF, 1998, 2000

[b]American Association of Clinical Endocrinologists (AACE). Clinical practice guidelines for the prevention and treatment of postmenopausal osteoporosis. Endocrinol Pract 1996;2(2):157–71.

useful if obtained prior to starting treatment and then repeated in 3 to 6 months to measure the response. Despite the fact that these markers may identify changes in bone remodeling, they do not predict fracture risk.

These tests are very expensive and are not recommended for screening or as the first-line studies to follow treatment response. However, if the BMD does not increase with treatment, one might order the turnover markers for further assessment.

Prevention and Treatment

Nonpharmacological

Nonpharmacological therapy for prevention and treatment of osteoporosis includes adequate dietary intake of calcium and vitamin D, weight-bearing exercise, fall precautions, no smoking, and avoidance of excessive alcohol intake. These steps should be started early in life and continued through menopause because BMD peaks at about age 35 and then begins to decline with accelerated bone loss after menopause.

Calcium

According to the National Institutes of Health (NIH) Consensus Development Conference, the optimal recommended dose of elemental calcium is the amount that each person needs to maintain adult bone mass and minimize bone loss later in life (Table 8.3). The recommended dose for postmenopausal women <65 years old who are on hormone replacement therapy (HRT) is 1000 mg/day and 1500 mg/day for all other postmenopausal women.[27] Calcium supplements are advisable if diet cannot supply the recommended amount necessary. Calcium citrate should be taken between meals while calcium carbonate should be taken with meals because it is best absorbed with gastric acid. Calcium should not be taken with iron because the iron decreases the absorption. Several studies show that calcium supplements can reduce bone loss in postmenopausal women and will reduce the risk of fractures.[27] The effect is not strong enough to recommend calcium alone for osteoporosis prevention.

Table 8.3. **Optimal Calcium Intake**

Population		NIH	RDA
Infants, children, and young adults			
0–6 Months		400	400
6–12 Months		600	600
1–10 years		800–1200	800
11–24 years		1200–1500	1200
Adult women			
Pregnant and lactating			
<24 years		1200–1500	1200
>24 years		1200	800
Premenopausal			
25–49 years		1000	800
Postmenopausal			
50–64 years	On estrogen	1000	800
	Not on estrogen	1500	800
≥65 years		1500	
Adult men			
25–64 years		1000	800
≥65 years		1500	800

[a]Calcium recommendations in mg/day.

NIH = National Institutes of Health; RDA = Recommended Daily Allowance.

Adapted from the NIH Consensus Conference, 1994.[18]

Vitamin D

The recommended daily intake of vitamin D needed for adequate calcium absorption is 400 to 800 IU. Vitamin D deficiency can occur in patients with inadequate sunlight exposure. Sunlight exposure is shown to be useful in preventing hip fractures, especially in elderly institutionalized women.[28]

Physical Activity

Adequate physical activity may exert a positive influence on bone mass and is necessary for bone acquisition and maintenance. The extent of this influence and the most effective type of program are not fully understood. Most trials of exercise intervention show that a reduction of falls is likely to be secondary to improved muscular strength and balance. Low-impact exercise like walking has minimal effect on BMD; high-impact exercise like weight training stimulates the increase of BMD. Women who exercise regularly are at a lower risk of hip fractures.[29] However, excessive exercise by competitive athletes can also be a risk factor for bone loss, particularly if they have hypoestrogenic oligo/amenorrhea.

Fall Prevention

Most osteoporotic fractures result from a fall. Risk factors for falling include visual or hearing problems, gait disturbances, underlying conditions that predispose the patient to syncope, cognitive impairment, and the use of certain medications such as diuretics, antihypertensive, benzodiazepines, and antidepressants. Home safety precautions may help to prevent falls. External hip protectors have been shown to provide protection against hip fractures in frail elderly adults.

Pharmacological Treatment

Pharmacological treatment should be initiated in women with:

No risk factors and who have T scores below 2 SDs
Risk factors and T scores below 1.5 SD
A history of vertebral or hip fractures
Multiple risk factors over 70 years of age without BMD measurement.

The pharmacological agents for treatment and prophylaxis of osteoporosis include HRT, calcium and vitamin D supplements, bisphosphonates, selective estrogen receptor modulators (SERMs), intranasal calcitonin, and parathyroid hormone (PTH). While the most widely prescribed regimen is HRT with calcium and vitamin D, there are many reasons to consider using the other medications.

Inhibitors of Bone Resorption

Hormonal

Hormone Replacement Therapy (HRT)

In the PEPI trial, HRT increased BMD at the hip by 1.7 % and at the spine by 3.5% to 5.0% over a 3-year period compared to placebo. HRT inhibits bone loss for the duration of the therapy, which recurs once therapy is discontinued. In premenopausal women with osteoporosis secondary to hypoestrogenic stages, early intervention with estrogen to achieve return of menses, is critical since bone loss may be irreversible.

Observational studies consistently suggest that postmenopausal HRT reduces the risk of hip and other types of fractures.[30] Evidence from randomized controlled trials (RCTs), especially for vertebral fracture prevention, is less available. In a Danish RCT, HRT reduced forearm fracture incidence in recent postmenopausal women.[31] In another randomized trial, HRT and vitamin D prevented nonvertebral fractures in postmenopausal women.[32] A meta-analysis published in 2001 suggests that estrogen reduces risk of nonvertebral fractures by 27%. Estrogen seemed to reduce the risk of fractures by 33% in younger women, but had no significant effect in women aged 60 years or older.[33]

Before starting a patient on HRT the physician and the patient need to consider all the risks and benefits. Common adverse effects such as breakthrough bleeding and breast tenderness or enlargement should be discussed. The risk of breast cancer and heart disease are very important issues. The relationship of HRT to breast cancer and heart disease is still controversial. HRT should be used with caution in patients who have a personal or family history of breast or endometrial cancer, or a history of a hypercoagulable state or thromboembolic episodes. Informed consent should be given to all patients.

In postmenopausal women without contraindications to HRT, any of the three recommended regimens could be used: estrogen alone in women without a uterus, estrogen with progestin daily, and estrogen with progestin in a cyclic manner (estrogen every day and progestin only for 10 to 14 days of the month). The most common regimen is conjugated estrogen at a daily dose of 0.625 mg or its equivalent. This dose can be used if the therapy begins at the onset of menopause in order to prevent the rapid bone loss that occurs early. If the postmenopausal woman is older at the time of starting the HRT, she might be more sensitive to the standard dose. One might consider starting at half the dose (0.3 mg) to avoid discontinuation secondary to adverse effects. Estrogen alone is avoided in women with a uterus in order to prevent endometrial cancer. Estrogen given with progesterone may actually decrease the risk of endometrial cancer.

Selective Estrogen Receptor Modulators (SERMs)

SERMs are an important alternative for women with contraindications or intolerance to estrogen therapy. Tamoxifen and raloxifene were FDA approved in 2000 for treatment of postmenopausal osteoporosis. The main goal is to maximize the beneficial estrogenic effect in bone and minimize the effect on the breast and endometrium.

One study showed that raloxifene may decrease the risk of vertebral fracture by 36%, but there has been no published evidence for hip fracture reduction.[34] Both SERMs are contraindicated in women at risk for deep venous thrombosis.

Bisphosphonates

Alendronate (Fosamax)

Alendronate was approved by the FDA in 1995 for treatment of postmenopausal osteoporosis. It reduces the risk of vertebral fractures by 30% to 50% and increases the BMD at the spine and hip.[35] Alendronate also reduces the risk of fractures in men and women with osteoporosis secondary to the chronic use of steroids.[36]

One study evaluated the addition of alendronate to HRT in the treatment of postmenopausal women with low BMD despite ongoing treatment with estrogen.[37] Compared with HRT alone, at 12 months alendronate plus HRT produced significantly greater increases in BMD of the lumbar spine (3.6% vs. 1.0%, $p < .001$) and hip trochanter (2.7% vs. 0.5%, $p < .001$). This study suggests that alendronate may be beneficial when added to HRT in postmenopausal women with low BMD despite ongoing treatment with HRT. However, it should be noted that the outcome measured was BMD and not fractures.

The recommended starting dose for postmenopausal osteoporosis prevention is 5 mg/day with a maintenance dose of 10 mg/day. The most common side effect is esophageal irritation secondary to reflux. Therefore, the patient should take alendronate with a full glass of water without food and remain upright for at least 30 minutes to avoid reflux. Another available regimen is 70 mg once a week. This weekly dose was demonstrated to be as effective with fewer gastrointestinal side effects.[38] At this time, the use of alendronate has not been approved for premenopausal women.

Risedronate (Actonel)

Risedronate is a newer biphosphonate approved in 2000 by the FDA for treatment of postmenopausal osteoporosis. While the indications are the same as alendronate, it has fewer gastrointestinal side effects. Both agents cost over $50 a month. In a randomized, double-blind, placebo-controlled trial of 2458 ambulatory postmenopausal women younger than 85 years with at least 1 vertebral fracture at baseline, risedronate decreased the relative incidence of new vertebral fractures by 41% over 3 years. The absolute risk reduction was from 16.3% to 11.3%. The cumulative incidence of nonvertebral fractures over 3 years was reduced by 39% (5.2 % vs 8.4%). The overall safety profile of risedronate, including gastrointestinal safety, was similar to that of placebo. The most effective dose was 5 mg/day.[39]

Calcitonin

Calcitonin is helpful when treating painful osteoporosis due to its significant analgesic effect. This hormone inhibits bone resorption by acting directly on the osteoclasts. The PROOF study is controversial; it demonstrates a reduction of vertebral fractures with calcitonin.[40] It is available in nasal spray at a recommended dose of 200 IU/day that corresponds to one squirt through one nostril every day alternating nostrils; or in the injectable form (200 units/mL) to be used three to five times/week at a dose of 50 to 100 IU/dose.

Stimulators of Bone Formation

Parathyroid Hormone (PTH)

PTH is the most promising anabolic agent that stimulates bone formation. It is still undergoing clinical trials. Even though it increases the BMD of the lumbar spine,[41] there are no data on fracture risk. One disadvantage is that it must be administered by subcutaneous injection. It is not yet approved by the FDA.

Fluoride

Fluoride stimulates bone formation but does not decrease the risk of a fracture. A meta-analysis showed that fluoride increases bone mineral density at the lumbar spine and does not reduce the number of vertebral fractures. Increasing the dose of fluoride actually increased the risk of nonvertebral fractures and gastrointestinal side effects.[42] It is not approved by the FDA for osteoporosis prevention and treatment.

Conclusion

Fractures of the hip, vertebrae, and wrists from osteoporosis cause significant decreases in the quality of life for many older individuals. The complications of hip fractures can also lead to death. Better methods for prevention, early detection, and treatment now exist. Healthy lifestyles, including no smoking, exercise, good diet, and calcium intake, can help to prevent osteoporosis. By assessing family history, ethnicity, body type, and other risk factors, physicians can target prevention and screening efforts to patients at highest risk for osteoporosis. Patients at higher risk should probably be screened using a DEXA scan. Pharmacological therapies such as hormone replacement, calcium, vitamin D, bisphosphonates, SERMs, and calcitonin can help prevent BMD loss and may reduce the risk of fractures. Currently, the data for fracture prevention are stronger for the bisphosponates than for hormonal therapy. Every family physician should feel comfortable screening for, preventing, and treating osteoporosis.

Suggested Web Sites

The National Institutes of Health Osteoporosis and Related Bone Diseases: National Resource Center *www.osteo.org*
The National Osteoporosis Foundation. *www.nof.org*

References

1. Riggs BL, Melton LJ III. The worldwide problem of osteoporosis: insights afforded by epidemiology. Bone 1995;17:505S–11S.
2. Chrischilles E, Shireman T, Wallace R. Costs and health effects of osteoporotic fractures. Bone 1994;15:377–87.
3. Lu Yao GL, Baron JA, Barrett JA. Treatment and survival among elderly Americans with hip fractures: a population-based study. Am J Public Health 1994;84:1287–91.
4. Watts NB. Hip fracture prevention in nursing homes: clinical importance and management strategies. Consult Pharm 1996;11:944–54.
5. Cummings SR, Kelsey JL, Nevitt MC. Epidemiology of osteoporosis and osteoporotic fractures. Epidemiol Rev 1985;7178–208.

6. Gold DT. The clinical impact of vertebral fractures. Bone 1996; 18:185–90.
7. World Health Organization (WHO) Study Group. Assessment of fracture risk and its application to screening for postmenopausal osteoporosis. Geneva, Switzerland: WHO Technical Report Series, 1994;843.
8. National Osteoporotic Foundation, 2025 osteoporosis prevalence figures: state by state report. January 1997. Women's Health Matters 1998; 2(30):1.
9. Harper KD, Weber TJ. Secondary osteoporosis. Diagnostic considerations. Endocrinol Metab Clin North Am 1998;27(2):325–48.
10. World Health Organization (WHO). Assessment of fracture risk and its application to screening for postmenopausal osteoporosis. WHO technical report series 843. Geneva: WHO, 1994.
11. Heinemann DF. Osteoporosis. An overview of the National Osteoporosis Foundation clinical practice guide. Geriatrics 2000;55(5):31–6.
12. Pocock NA, Eisman JA, Hopper JL. Genetic determinants of bone mass in adults. J Clin Invest 1987;80:706–10.
13. Seeman E. Growth in bone mass and size: are racial and gender differences in bone density more apparent than real? J Clin Endocrinol Metab 1998;83:1414–18.
14. Harper KD, Weber TJ. Secondary osteoporosis. Diagnostic considerations. Endocrinol Metab Clin North Am 1998;27(2):325–48.
15. Saag KG, Emkey R, Schinitzer A. For the glucocorticoid-induced osteoporosis intervention study group. Alendronate for the prevention and treatment of glucocorticoid-induced osteoporosis. N Engl J Med 1998;339:292–9.
16. Bassey EJ, Rothwell MC, Littlewood JJ. Pre- and post-menopausal women have different bone mineral density responses to the same high impact exercise. J Bone Miner Res 1998;13:1805–13.
17. Dawson B, Harris SS, Krall EA. Effect of calcium and vitamin D supplementation on bone density in men and women 65 years of age or older. N Engl J Med 1997;337:670–6.
18. NIH Consensus Development Panel on Optimal Calcium Intake. NIH Consensus Conference: optimal calcium intake. JAMA 1994;272: 1942–8.
19. Hotta M, Shibasaki T, Sato K. The importance of body weight history in the occurrence and recovery of osteoporosis in patients with anorexia nervosa: evaluation by dual x-ray absorptiometry and bone metabolic markers. Eur J Endocrinol 1998;139:276–83.
20. Consensus Development Conference. Diagnosis, prophylaxis and treatment of osteoporosis. Am J Med 1993;94:646–50.
21. Nattiv A. Osteoporosis: its prevention, recognition, and management. Family Pract Recert 1998;20(2):17–41.
22. Black DM, Cummings SR, Genant HK. Axial and appendicular bone density predict fractures in older women. J Bone Miner Res 1996;11:707–30.
23. AACE Clinical Practice guidelines for the prevention and treatment of postmenopausal osteoporosis. Endocrinol Pract 1996;2(2):157–71.

24. National Osteoporosis Foundation. Physicians guide to prevention and treatment of osteoporosis. Bele Mead, NJ: Experta Medica, 1998.
25. NIH Consensus Conference. Osteoporosis prevention, diagnosis and therapy. JAMA 2001;285(6):785–94.
26. Garnero P, Hauserr E, Chapui MC. Markers of bone resorption predict hip fracture in elderly women: the EPIDOS prospective study. J Bone Miner Res 1996;11:1531–8.
27. Reid R, Ames RW, Evans MC. Effect of calcium supplementation on bone loss in postmenopausal women. N Engl J Med 1993;328:460–4.
28. Chapuy MC, Arlot ME, Duboeuf F. Vitamin D3 and calcium to prevent hip fractures in the elderly women. N Engl J Med 1992;327:1637–42.
29. Paganini-Hill A, Chao A, Ross RK. Exercise and other factors in the prevention of hip fracture: the Leisure World study. Epidemiology 1991;2:16–25.
30. Grady D, Cummings SR. Postmenopausal hormone therapy for prevention of fractures: how good is the evidence? JAMA 2001;285(22): 2909–10.
31. Mosekilde L, Beck-Nielsen H, Sorensen OH, et al. Hormonal replacement therapy reduces forearm fracture incidence in recent postmenopausal women—results of the Danish Osteoporosis Prevention Study. Maturitas 2000;36(3):181–93.
32. Komulainen MH, Kroger H, Tuppurainen MT, et al. HRT and Vit D in prevention of non-vertebral fractures in postmenopausal women; a 5 year randomized trial. Maturitas. 1998;31(1):45–54.
33. Torgerson DJ, Bell-Syer SEM. Hormone replacement therapy and prevention of nonvertebral fractures: a meta-analysis of randomized trials. JAMA 2001;285:2891–7.
34. Ettinger B, Black DM, Mitlak BH. Reduction of vertebral fracture risk in postmenopausal women with osteoporosis treated with raloxifene: results from a 3-year randomized clinical trial. JAMA 1999;282:637–45.
35. Karpf DB, Shapiro DR, Seeman E. Prevention of nonvertebral fractures by alendronate: a meta-analysis. JAMA 1997;277:1159–64.
36. Saag KG, Emkey R, Schnitzer TJ, et al. Alendronate for the prevention and treatment of glucocorticoid-induced osteoporosis. Glucocorticoid-Induced Osteoporosis Intervention Study Group. N Engl J Med 1998;339(5):292–9.
37. Lindsay R, Cosman F, Lobo RA, et al. Addition of alendronate to ongoing hormone replacement therapy in the treatment of osteoporosis: a randomized, controlled clinical trial. J Clin Endocrinol Metab 1999;84(9):3076–81.
38. Baran D. Osteoporosis. Efficacy and safety of a bisphosphonate dosed once weekly. Geriatrics 2001;56(3):28–32.
39. Harris ST, Watts NB, Genant HK. Effects of risedronate treatment on vertebral and nonvertebral fractures in women with postmenopausal osteoporosis. JAMA 1999;282:1344–52.
40. Chestnut CH, Silverman SL, Andriano K. Salmon calcitonin nasal spray reduces the rate of new vertebral fractures independently of known major pre-treatment risk factors: accrued 5 year analysis of the PROOF study. Bone 1998;23(5):S290.

41. Lindsay R, Cosman F, Nieves J. Does treatment with parathyroid hormone increases vertebral size? Osteoporosis International 2000. World Congress on Osteoporosis 2000;11(2):556,S206.
42. Haguenauer D, Welch V, Shea B, Tugwell P, Adachi JD, Wells G. Fluoride for the treatment of postmenopausal osteoporotic fractures: a meta-analysis. Osteoporos Int 2000;11(9):727–38.

9
Gout

James F. Calvert, Jr.

Gout encompasses a spectrum of diseases caused by precipitation of uric acid crystals in tissue. The gouty disorders include (1) acute monarticular arthritis caused by uric acid crystals in joints, (2) nephrolithiasis, (3) soft tissue deposits of urate crystals known as tophi, and (4) uric acid renal disease. Gout occurs in about 1.3% of men over 40, making it the most common form of inflammatory arthritis in men. The prevalence in women is about half that in men,[1] although there is evidence that the relative prevalence of gout in women has increased.[2] The prevalence of gout increases with age, and it is more common in persons of African or Polynesian ancestry.

Hyperuricemia

Hyperuricemia is caused by either increased production of uric acid or decreased ability to excrete it; some of the more common disorders characterized by hyperuricemia are listed in Table 9.1. Hyperuricemia is defined as the presence of a serum uric acid over 7.0 mg/dL (420 μmol/L). Uric acid is less likely to form crystals at concentrations below this level. The risk of having all the gouty disorders increases proportionately to the serum uric acid level.[3] Prophylactic treatment to lower the uric acid level incurs no benefit to patients with asymptomatic hyperuricemia and is more risky and expensive than no treatment,[4] although the discovery that a patient has hyperuricemia should lead to an attempt to determine its etiology and significance. An exception to this rule is that patients with lymphoproliferative disorders or those about to undergo chemotherapy for other malignancies should be treated prophylactically with allopurinol.[5,6] Uric acid levels

Table 9.1. **Some Possible Causes of Hyperuricemia**

Endogenous causes
  Family history
  Overproduction or underexcretion of urate
  Large body build
  Rapid cell turnover (malignancy)
  Renal failure
  Hypertension
Exogenous causes
  Dietary purine: organ meats, kale, spinach, shellfish, beans
  Alcohol, especially beer
  Medications: especially diuretics and antimetabolites (e.g.,
    cyclosporine)
  Poisons: lead, others

are often elevated prior to the development of heart disease, stroke, hyperlipidemia, diabetes, and hyperinsulinism, but whether the hyperuricemia is an innocent bystander in these disorders or part of their cause is a matter of controversy.[7–9]

Acute Gout

Acute gout is characterized by severe pain in a single joint that develops over a period of a few hours. Uric acid is more likely to crystalize at lower temperatures, so the metatarsophalangeal joint of the great toe, the coolest part of the body, is the most common site of gouty attacks, but other joints, typically a knee, shoulder, hand, or another part of the foot or ankle, are the site of presentation in 30% to 50% of cases.[10] Gout can present in any joint, and the inflammation can be extremely subtle in some cases; hence a search for crystals should be undertaken for all arthritis of unknown etiology. More than half of women with gout have polyarticular disease,[11] a presentation that is also common in the elderly. Chronic gout is uncommon but does occur, most often in postmenopausal women. Attacks of acute gout commonly follow trauma or surgery, especially in patients with hyperuricemia.

Diagnosis of Acute Gout

With acute oligoarticular gout the skin over the affected joint is usually red and warm; peeling of the skin is common, and pain is typically so severe the patient does not allow anything to touch the affected joint. Low-grade fever, elevated peripheral white blood cell

(WBC) count, and elevated erythrocyte sedimentation rate (ESR) are commonly seen in patients with acute gout. Because of these characteristics the appearance of acute oligoarticular gout is distinctive, and the most important item in the differential diagnosis is joint infection. This distinction can be particularly troublesome in the hand.[12]

Diagnostic Studies

The serum uric acid level is not helpful for excluding or confirming a diagnosis of gout. Although clinical diagnostic criteria have been developed for acute gout, examination of synovial fluid under polarized light provides the only definitive diagnosis.[13] Acute synovitis due to deposition of pyrophosphate crystals (pseudogout) becomes more common after age 65, so joint aspiration is particularly important for this age group.

Synovial fluid can easily be obtained by passing an 18-gauge or smaller needle into the joint and aspirating it. Many clinicians prefer to numb the surrounding soft tissue with lidocaine before attempting joint entry. Joint fluid is then sent for crystal examination, cell count, Gram stain, and culture. The cell count is over 20,000/cu mL in those with gout or infection, and counts as high as 100,000/cu mL may be seen with either; the presence of crystals is the only reliable indicator that gout rather than infection is present. The needle-shaped crystals of gout have a unique appearance under polarized light; they are about the size of a neutrophil and are commonly seen inside them. In patients with acute gout the joint radiographs may be normal, but the erosions seen with chronic gout are fairly specific and can be helpful in making that diagnosis (Fig. 9.1). Radiographs can help identify unsuspected fractures or osteomyelitis in patients with acute arthritis.[14]

Treatment of Gout and Hyperuricemia

Treatment of gout specifically addresses one of three clinical entities: (1) acute gout, (2) the intercritical period that occurs for 2 to 3 months after an acute attack, or (3) long-term management of chronic hyperuricemia.

Treatment of Acute Gout

Attacks of acute gout are most commonly managed by nonsteroidal antiinflammatory drugs (NSAIDs) (see Chapter 4). High doses are needed. Although all NSAIDs are probably effective for acute gout,

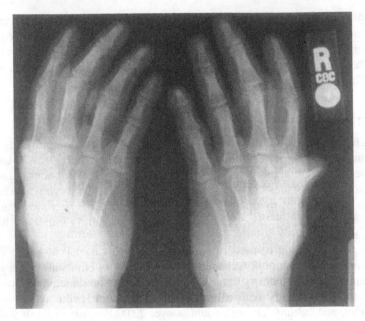

Fig. 9.1. Radiograph of the hand of a patient with gout. There are typical margin erosions and areas of radiolucency at the proximal interphalangeal joints of the index and long fingers bilaterally.

indomethacin (Indocin) is commonly used. One regimen involves giving indomethacin 50 mg four times a day for the first 2 days, then 50 mg three times a day for a week, then 50 mg twice a day for a week, then 25 mg two or three times a day for 2 to 3 weeks (or more). Acute gout can also be treated with colchicine in a dose of 0.6 mg/hr by mouth up to a total of 5 or 6 mg until relief or severe gastrointestinal side effects occur. At one time it was thought that colchicine was effective only for acute gouty arthritis, and so its use had utility in the differential diagnosis; it is now known that colchicine is at times successful for any form of acute arthritis.[15] Colchicine can be given intravenously, a method that reduces side effects; but the drug is potentially toxic in this form, and it is recommended that physicians considering the use of intravenous colchicine carefully review the instructions for its use.[16] For patients who are unlikely to tolerate treatment with NSAIDs or colchicine (e.g., those with gastrointestinal disease or renal failure), intraarticular or even systemic steroids can be used. Another option is the use of a single dose of 60 mg of depo-triamcinolone (Kenalog) intramuscularly.[17] Adrenocorticotropic hormone (ACTH) is also effective in a dose of 0.4 mg (40 units) IM, which may have to be repeated every 12 hours for 2 to 3 days.[13,18]

Management of Intercritical Gout

Patients who have had resolution of an acute gouty attack are susceptible to a recurrence in the same joint for the next 2 to 3 months, a period known as the intercritical period. Hence, preventive therapy is indicated for several months after an acute attack. Oral colchicine at 0.6 mg one or two times a day is effective for this purpose and is unlikely to have any side effects. Low-dose colchicine can be started along with NSAIDs at the time of an acute attack. Another alternative is low-dose NSAID therapy, such as indomethacin 25 mg twice a day, though this alternative is more likely to cause side effects.

Hypouricemic agents (e.g., allopurinol or probenecid) worsen an acute gouty attack and are never used during one. After some weeks of intercritical treatment the possibility of starting chronic drug therapy to lower the serum uric acid level can be considered. In patients who have only an occasional gouty attack and have no complication of gout such as tophi or gouty renal disease (see section below), treatment of hyperuricemia is optional; some patients prefer the risk of an occasional attack to taking medicine on a long-term basis. Patients who believe their attacks are frequent enough to justify treatment or in whom treatment is indicated because of tophi or gouty renal disease should undergo treatment directed at hyperuricemia. Most experts believe that dietary therapy is of marginal benefit in lowering uric acid levels,[19] although patients should be advised to lose weight and reduce consumption of alcohol, meats, fat, and cholesterol. Hydration is important. Avoidance of medications that elevate the serum uric acid level is also helpful. Low-dose aspirin, niacin, and diuretics are the most common of these agents, and cyclosporine is another offender.

Hyperuricemia

Medical treatment of hyperuricemia involves use of either uricosuric agents or allopurinol (Zyloprim), an agent that interferes with uric acid metabolism. The choice of agent depends on patient characteristics. Allopurinol is indicated in patients with nephrolithiasis, tophi, or renal disease. It is also indicated in patients with congenital overproduction of uric acid. These patients can be identified by collecting a 24-hour urine specimen for uric acid assay; the uric acid content is more than 1 g in overproducers (some clinicians use 600 or 800 mg as the cutoff).

Patients with hyperuricemia who excrete less than 1 g/24 hr are considered to be underexcreters and can be treated with a uricosuric agent instead of allopurinol unless they have nephrolithiasis, tophi, or renal failure. Probenecid (Benemid), the most commonly used uricosuric agent, is started at 250 mg twice a day for a few days, then increased to 500 mg twice a day, and gradually increased up to a total of 3 g/day if needed. The goal of therapy is to get the serum uric acid below 6.0 mg/dL (360 μmol/L), although a level of 5 mg/dL (300 μmol/L) or less more effectively dissolves uric acid crystals. Gastric intolerance to probenecid is fairly common, and many drug interactions occur; for example, aspirin eliminates the uricosuric effect of probenecid. The cost of probenecid is also slightly higher than that of allopurinol. For this reason, many clinicians prefer to use allopurinol even in underexcreters. It is effective against any form of hyperuricemia.

Allopurinol should be started at a dose of 100 mg/day and increased gradually up to 300 mg/day if needed to keep the serum uric acid under 6.0 mg/dL (360 μmol/L). If the serum uric acid remains elevated in a patient on allopurinol 300 mg/day, noncompliance should be suspected,[20] although doses up to 800 mg/day are occasionally needed. The most common side effect of allopurinol is a rash; a vasculitic syndrome affecting the skin and kidneys accompanied by fever, leukocytosis, eosinophilia, and hepatitis may be seen. This syndrome is more common among the elderly and in patients with renal failure or on diuretic therapy; in these patients use of the lowest possible dose of allopurinol and a goal of 7 mg/dL (420 μmol/L) rather than 6 mg/dL (360 μmol/L) can be considered. When this syndrome occurs, it is treated with high-dose steroids.

Acute attacks of gout are common when either uricosuric agents or allopurinol are started, even if several months have elapsed since the patient's last attack. It is important to warn patients of this possibility. Continuing prophylactic therapy with colchicine at 0.6 mg once or twice a day for the first year of hypouricemic therapy is advised. Starting with low doses of hypouricemic agents, as noted above, is also helpful. Urate-lowering drugs should not be started until a month has passed since the last acute attack of gout, and, if possible, colchicine should be started first and continued for the first few months of treatment with urate-lowering therapy, although the risk of possible toxicity to colchicine needs to be considered.[13]

Finally, patient education is an important component in the management of gout. Patients need to understand the difference between the agents used to control acute gout, the intercritical period, and chronic therapy with urate-lowering agents, or there will be substantial confusion and worsening of their condition.[20] Patients need to be followed regularly by the same provider with frequent monitoring of their uric acid levels for those on urate-lowering therapy; patient education can occur during these visits.

Uric Acid Nephropathy

Uric acid nephropathy is caused by precipitation of uric acid crystals in the renal tubules. It is usually due to a sudden overproduction of uric acid in a dehydrated patient (e.g., following vigorous exercise).[21] Uric acid nephropathy can also be seen in patients with aggressive leukemia or during chemotherapy leading to rapid cell turnover. Uric acid nephropathy can be treated with vigorous hydration, diuretics, and alkalinization of urine; prevention is often possible if patients at risk are kept well hydrated.

Tophi

Tophi are aggregates of uric acid crystals surrounded by a giant cell foreign-body reaction. They gradually enlarge with time and eventually become first radiopaque and then obvious on physical examination. They appear around joints and in the subcutaneous tissues. Their presence is an indication for allopurinol therapy, which gradually leads to their dissolution. Tophi are much less common now than previously, probably because hyperuricemia is treated more aggressively.[13]

Pseudogout

Arthritis due to deposition of calcium pyrophosphate dihydrate, or calcium pyrophosphate deposition disease (CPDD), is often called pseudogout. The knee is the most commonly affected joint; the disease is much more common in the elderly. Radiographs show chondrocalcinosis. The diagnosis is made by synovial fluid analysis; the joint fluid is similar to that seen in gout except that the crystals are characteristic. Treatment of an acute attack is the same as that for acute gout, and colchicine prophylaxis can prevent recurrence.

References

1. Peacock DJ, Cooper C. Epidemiology of the rheumatic diseases. Curr Opin Rheumatol 1995;7(2):82–6.
2. Gabriel SE. Update on the epidemiology of the rheumatic diseases. Curr Opin Rheumatol 1996;8(2):96–100.

3. Harris MD, Siegel LB, Alloway JA. Gout and hyperuricemia. Am Fam Physician 1999;59(4):925–34.
4. Campion EW, Glynn RJ, DeLarby DO. Asymptomatic hyperuricemia: risks and consequences in the Normative Aging Study. Am J Med 1987;82:421–6.
5. Van Doomum S, Ryan PFJ. Clinical manifestations of gout and their management. Med J Aust 2000;172:493–7.
6. Davis JC. A practical approach to gout. Postgrad Med 1999;106(4): 115–23.
7. Berkowitz D. Gout, hyperlipidemia, and diabetes interrelationships. JAMA 1966;197:41:227–42.
8. Johnson RJ, Kivlighn SD, Kim Y, et al. Reappraisal of the pathogenesis and consequences of hyperuricemia in hypertension, cardiovascular disease, and renal disease. Am J Kidney Dis 1999;33(2):225–34.
9. Pittman JR, Bross MH. Diagnosis and management of gout. Am Fam Physician 1999;59(7):1799–806.
10. Snaith ML. Gout, hyperuricemia, and crystal arthritis. BMJ 1995;310: 521–4.
11. Joseph J, McGrath H. Gout or 'pseudogout': how to differentiate crystal-induced arthropathies. Geriatrics 1995;50(4):13–39.
12. Louis DS, Jebson DL. Mimickers of hand infections. Hand Clin 1998;14(4):519–29.
13. Fam AG. Managing problem gout. Ann Acad Med Singapore 1998;27: 93–9.
14. Beutler A, Schumacher HR. Gout and 'pseudogout': when are arthritic symptoms caused by crystal deposition? Postgrad Med 1994;2:103–20.
15. Ben-Chetrit E, Micha L. Colchicine: 1998 update. Semin Arthritis Rheum 1998;28(1):48–59.
16. Milne ST, Meek PD. Fatal colchicine overdose: report of a case and review of the literature. Am J Emerg Med 1998;16(6):603–8.
17. Alloway JA, Moriarty MJ, Hoogland YT, et al. Comparison of triamcinolone acetonide with indomethacin in the treatment of acute gouty arthritis. J Rheumatol 1993;20:1383–5.
18. Axelrod D, Preston D. A comparison of parenteral adrenocorticotrophic hormone with indomethacin in the treatment of acute gout. Arthritis Rheum 1988;31:803–5.
19. Emmerson BT. The management of gout. N Engl J Med 1996;334(7): 445–51.
20. Corkill MM. Gout. NZ Med J 1994;107:337–9.
21. Wortmann RL. Effective management of gout: an analogy. Am J Med 1998;105:513–14.

10
Athletic Injuries

Michael L. Tuggy and Cora Collette Breuner

Family physicians routinely treat many athletic injuries in their clinical practice. The benefits of long-term exercise in the prevention of common illnesses such as cardiovascular disease, osteoporosis, and falls in the elderly are well established. With the increased interest in fitness in the general population, the number of people resuming more active exercise as they age is increasing. Injuries sustained in childhood or adolescence may have long-term effects that can hamper later attempts at physical activity.[1] For all ages of patients, proper training and prevention can lead to lifelong participation in athletic activities.

Most sports injuries are related to overuse injuries and often are not brought to the attention of the family physician until the symptoms are advanced. Traumatic injuries are more readily diagnosed, but may have more serious long-term sequelae for the life of the athlete. Sport selection has a great impact on risk of injury. The adolescent athlete is probably at highest risk for injury due to sport selection, presence of immature growth cartilage at the growth plates and joint surfaces, and lack of experience.[2] High-risk sports selected by young adults also have higher degrees of risk, which can be modified to lessen injury rates by training and education. Table 10.1 lists common sports activities and their relative injury rates.

Mechanisms of Injury

Direct trauma is a common mechanism that leads to injury. Deceleration injuries are the most common form of serious injury,

Table 10.1. **Common Sports Injuries and Injury Rates**

Sports activity	Common injuries	Injury rate (per 1000 exposures)
Running	Tibial periostitis, stress fracture Metatarsal stress fractures	14
Football	ACL/MCL tears Shoulder dislocation/ separation Ankle sprain	13
Wrestling	Shoulder dislocation MCL, LCL tears	12
Gymnastics	Spondylolysis/spondylolisthesis Ankle sprains	10
Alpine/telemark skiing	ACL/MCL tears Skier's thumb Shoulder dislocation	9
Basketball	Ankle sprains Shoulder dislocation/separation	4
Baseball	Lateral epicondylitis Rotator cuff tear	4
Cross-country skiing	Ankle sprains Lateral epicondylitis	3

ACL = anterior cruciate ligament; LCL = lateral collateral ligament; MCL = medial collateral ligament.

resulting in significant blunt trauma or joint injury. The athlete's momentum, enhanced by self-generated speed, gravity, and equipment, is translated into energy when impact occurs. This energy is then absorbed by the body in the form of blunt trauma, torsion of joints, or transfer of stress within the skeleton.

Collision sports, such as football or rugby, and high-velocity sports, such as alpine skiing, have much higher rates of significant musculoskeletal injury due to the combination of speed and mass effect on impact. Factors that affect the extent of injury include tensile strength of the ligaments and tendons of affected joints, bony strength, flexibility, and ability of the athlete to reduce the impact. This is where appropriate conditioning for a sport reduces injury risk. Not only are endurance and strength training important, but also practicing falls or recovery from falls can help the athlete diffuse the energy of the fall or impact. Athletes should be encouraged to use the appropriate safety equipment and to train comprehensively for their sport.

Overuse injuries comprise the most common form of sports injuries seen by the family physician. These injuries are induced by repetitive motion leading to microscopic disruption of a bone–tendon or bone–synovium interface. This microtrauma initiates an inflammatory response. If the inflammatory response is not modulated by a rest phase or is excessive due to mechanical factors, then degradation of the tendon or bone may occur. Predisposing factors that lead to overuse injuries include poor flexibility, imbalance of strength of opposing muscle groups, mechanical deformity (e.g., pes planus), inadequate rest between exercise periods, and faulty equipment.[3] Adolescent athletes are especially vulnerable to such injuries, especially in areas where growth cartilage is present in the epiphyseal or apophyseal attachments of major muscle groups. Elderly athletes also are at higher risk because of preexisting degenerative joint disease (DJD) and poor flexibility.

Overuse injuries can be classified in four stages. Stage 1 injuries are symptomatic only during vigorous exercise and stage 2 during moderate exercise. Stage 3 injuries are symptomatic during minimal exercise, and the symptoms usually last up to 24 hours after exercise has ceased. Stage 4 injuries are painful at rest with no exercise to exacerbate the symptoms. Most overuse injuries are seen at later stages by physicians (stage 3 or 4) and require significant alteration in training schedules to allow healing of the injury. Progressive inflammation from overuse can eventually lead to tendon disruption, periostitis (stress reaction), true stress fractures, or cartilaginous degeneration. Early periostitis may only appear as a "fluffiness" of the cortical margin with compensatory cortical thickening underlying it (Fig. 10.1). In more advanced cases, the margin is clearly blurred and the cortex significantly thickened. If symptoms suggest a significant stress reaction but x-rays are negative, then a bone scan is indicated. True stress fractures can be visualized on plain film while stress reactions (periostitis) are best seen on bone scan. Because stress fractures are inflammatory in nature, the complication rates due to delayed or nonunion are higher than those with traumatic fractures.[4] The results of improper treatment of these injuries can be severe, resulting in permanent degenerative changes or deformity. The primary care provider plays an important role not only in diagnosing the injury early (and thus shortening the rehabilitation period) but also in stressing prevention with proper training guidance and timely intervention.

Traumatic Injuries

Physicians providing coverage for athletic events must recognize high-risk situations for serious injuries and evaluate the safety of the sports environment. Asking the following questions when first evaluating a patient with a traumatic injury helps suggest the correct

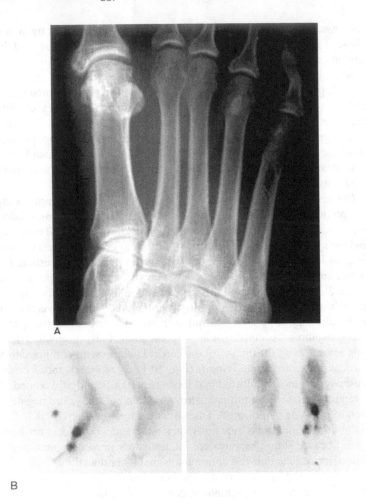

Fig. 10.1. (A) Periostitis of the proximal second metatarsal characterized by thickening of the cortex and "fluffy" appearance of the medial margin of the cortex. (B) The confirmatory bone scan identified two areas of significant inflammation of the second metatarsal.

diagnosis and focus the physical examination. During what sport did the injury occur? How did the injury occur? Where does it hurt? What aggravates the pain? Did other symptoms accompany the injury? Did swelling occur and if so, how soon? How old is the athlete? Has the athlete been injured before? Once these questions are answered, the physician should then perform a focused musculoskeletal and neurovascular exam.

Ankle Injuries

Ankle injuries are ubiquitous and constitute the most common acute musculoskeletal injury, affecting the entire spectrum of grade school to professional athletes. It is estimated that 1 million people present with ankle injuries each year, with an average cost of $300 to $900 for diagnosis and rehabilitation requiring 36 to 72 days for complete rehabilitation. Basketball players have the highest rate of ankle injuries, followed by football players and cross-country runners.[5] Eighty-five percent of athletes with ankle sprains have inversion injuries. The most common structures injured with inversion are the three lateral ligaments that support the ankle joint: the anterior and posterior talofibular ligaments, and the calcaneofibular ligament (Fig. 10.2). The other primary mechanism of ankle sprains is eversion, accounting for 15% of ankle injuries. In general, these are more severe than inversion injuries because of a higher rate of fractures and disruptions of the ankle mortise, leading to instability. The deltoid ligament is the most common ligament to be injured in eversion injuries. Fifteen percent of all complete ligament tears are associated with avulsion fractures of the tibia, fibula, talus, or the base of the fifth metatarsal. Epiphyseal growth plate injuries may be present in the young athlete who sustains

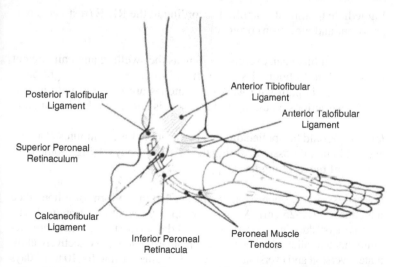

Fig. 10.2. Lateral view of major ankle ligaments and structures.

an ankle injury. Clinical evidence for an epiphyseal injury of the distal fibula or tibia is bony tenderness about two finger breadths proximal to the tip of the malleolus.[6]

Diagnosis

The examination in the immediate postinjury period may be limited by swelling, pain, and muscle spasm. Inspection should focus on an obvious deformity and vascular integrity. Ankle x-rays are necessary only if there is inability to bear weight for four steps both immediately and in the emergency department, or if there is bony tenderness at the posterior edge or tip of either malleoli.[7] The patient should be reexamined after the swelling has subsided, as the second examination may be more useful in pinpointing areas of tenderness. A pain-free passive and active range of motion of the ankle should be determined in all aspects of movement. The anterior drawer test should be used to assess for joint instability. A positive test, which entails the palpable and visible displacement of the foot more than 4 mm out of the mortise, is consistent with a tear of the anterior talofibular ligament and the anterior joint capsule.[8] Injuries to the lateral ligament complex are assigned grades 1, 2, or 3 depending on the amount of effusion and functional disability.

Management

Immediate treatment is applied according to the RICE (rest, ice, compression, and elevation) protocol.

Rest. The athlete can exercise as long as the swelling and pain are not worse within 24 hours. Exercise should include simple weight bearing. If there is pain with walking, crutches are required with appropriate instructions on use until the athlete is able to walk without pain.

Ice. Ice should be applied directly to the ankle for 20 minutes at a time every 2 hours, if possible, during the first 1 to 2 days. Icing should continue until the swelling has stopped.

Compression. Compression can be applied in the form of a horseshoe felt adhesive (0.625 cm). An elastic wrap will do but is not optimal. The compression dressing is worn for 2 to 3 days. Air stirrup braces are recommended to allow dorsiflexion and plantar flexion and effectively eliminate inversion and eversion. For grade 3 sprains, casting for 10 to 14 days may be an option.

Elevation. The leg should be elevated as much as possible until the swelling has stabilized.

Orthopedic Referral

Indications for orthopedic referral include the following factors: fracture, dislocation, evidence of neurovascular compromise, penetrating wound into the joint space, and grade 3 sprain with tendon rupture. All patients with ankle injuries should begin early rehabilitation exercises, including passive range of motion and graduated strength training immediately after the injury.

Overview of Knee Injuries

It has been estimated that during each week of the fall football season at least 6000 high school and college players injure their knees, 10% of whom require surgery.[9] Even more discouraging are the results of a 20-year follow-up study of men who had sustained a knee injury in high school. The investigators found that 39% of the men continued to have significant symptoms, 50% of whom had radiographic abnormalities.[9] Knee braces, while popular, have not been proven to be effective in preventing knee ligament injuries. The best time to evaluate the knee is immediately after the injury. Within an hour of a knee injury, protective muscle spasm can prevent a reliable assessment of the joint instability. The following day there may be enough joint effusion to preclude a satisfactory examination. When evaluating knee injuries, compare the injured knee to the uninjured knee. The Pittsburgh Decision Rules delineate evidence-based guidelines for when radiographs should be obtained. In general, any sports injury that involves a fall or torsional stress to the knee resulting in an effusion would mandate a knee radiograph. Knee radiographs are necessary to rule out tibial eminence fractures, epiphyseal fractures, and osteochondral fractures. Finally, an evaluation of the neurovascular status of the leg and foot is mandatory.

Meniscus Injuries

Meniscus injuries can occur from twisting or rotation of the knee along with deep flexion and hyperextension. Symptoms include pain, recurrent effusions, clicking, and with associated limited range of motion. Meniscus flaps may become entrapped within the joint space, resulting in locking or the knee "giving out."

Diagnosis

Classically, meniscus tears are characterized by tenderness or pain over the medial or lateral joint line either in hyperflexion or hyperextension. This should be differentiated from tenderness along the entire medial collateral ligament elicited when that ligament is sprained. When the lower leg is rotated with the knee flexed about 90 degrees, pain during external rotation indicates a medial meniscus injury (McMurray's test).

Management

After a meniscus injury, the athlete should follow the RICE protocol. Crutch usage should be insisted upon to avoid weight bearing until the pain and edema have diminished. In most athletes, an orthopedic referral should be considered for arthroscopy in order to repair the damaged meniscus. Plan for follow-up to initiate a rehabilitative program and return to sports.

Medial Collateral Ligament (MCL) Sprain

The MCL ligament is the medial stabilizer of the knee and it is usually injured by an excessive valgus stress of the knee. The resulting stress can result in a first-, second-, or third-degree sprain. MCL tears are often associated with medial meniscus injury. Lateral collateral ligament tears are unusual and are caused by an inwardly directed blow (varus force) to the inside of the knee.

Diagnosis

The player is usually able to bear some weight on the leg immediately after the injury. Medial knee pain is usually felt at the time of the injury and the knee may feel "wobbly" while the player walks afterward. The examination will reveal acute tenderness somewhere over the course of the MCL usually at or above the joint line. The integrity of the MCL is assessed by applying a valgus stress to the knee while holding the tibia about a third of the way down and forcing it gently laterally while holding the distal femur in place. A patient with a partial (grade 1 or 2) tear of a collateral ligament will have marked discomfort with valgus and varus testing. The athlete with a complete (grade 3) tear of a collateral ligament may have surprisingly little pain on testing but remarkably increased laxity of the ligament. Swelling, ecchymosis over the ligament or a joint effusion, usually develops within several hours of the injury.

Management

A grade 1 sprain is treated with the RICE protocol. Running should be restricted until the athlete is pain free in knee flexion. Generally in 5 to 10 days there will be complete recovery, and with physician clearance, the player can resume full activity. The management of more serious sprains should be directed by an orthopedist.

Anterior Cruciate Ligament (ACL) Injury

This is the most frequent and most severe ligament injury to the knee. It usually occurs not with a direct blow to the knee, but rather from torsional stress coupled with a deceleration injury. These injuries are seen when an athlete changes direction while running and the knee suddenly "gives out."

Diagnosis

A "pop" is often felt during the injury. The player falls on the field in extreme pain and is unable to continue participating. A bloody effusion will develop in 60% to 70% of athletes within the next 24 hours. One of three tests can be employed to test for ACL insufficiency: the anterior drawer, the Lachman maneuver, or the pivot shift test. The *anterior drawer test* should be performed with the knee in 30 degrees of flexion. The injured leg is externally rotated slightly to relax the hamstrings and adductor muscles. The examiner kneels lateral to the injured leg, stabilizes the femur with one hand, and directs a gentle but firm upward force with the other hand on the proximal tibia. If the tibia moves anteriorly, then the ACL has been torn. The *Lachman test* is performed with the hamstrings relaxed and the knee placed in 15 to 20 degrees of flexion. With one hand on the femur just above the knee to stabilize it, the tibia is pulled forward with the opposite hand placed over the tibial tuberosity. If the ACL is intact, the tibia comes to a firm stop. If the ligament is torn the tibia continues forward sluggishly. A *pivot shift test* is performed with the ankle and leg held under the examiner's arm. The leg is abducted and the knee extended. Place the knee in internal rotation with gentle valgus stress to the knee. The hands are placed under the proximal tibia while the knee is flexed to about 25 degrees. If the lateral tibial condyle rotates anteriorly (subluxes forward) during the flexion maneuver, then the test is positive.

Posterior cruciate ligament injuries are usually caused by a direct blow to the upper anterior tibia or posterior forces applied to the tibia while the knee is in flexion. This might apply to a karate player who is kicked in the area of the tibial tuberosity while the foot is firmly on the ground, or to someone who falls forward onto a flexed knee. Posterior cruciate ligament tears are detected by posterior displacement of the tibial tuberosity (the *sag sign*) when the leg is held by the heel with the hip and knee flexed.

Management

Initial management of ACL tears follows the RICE protocol along with immobilization and crutches, with instructions on their use. The rehabilitation requires the early initiation of quadriceps contractions to prevent atrophy and promote strengthening. Protective bracing with a hinged knee brace may be appropriate for certain athletes. Referral to an orthopedist should be made acutely if there is evidence on x-ray of an avulsion fracture of the ACL attachments or subacutely for possible arthroscopic repair if there is joint laxity.

Patellar Dislocation

This injury can result from a blow to the patella or when an athlete changes direction and then straightens the leg. It is most common in athletes with significant valgus deformity of the knee joint and in adolescents.

Diagnosis

The dislocation usually occurs laterally, but the medial joint capsule and retinaculum may also be torn, sometimes simulating or actually associated with a medial collateral ligament sprain. The dislocation usually reduces spontaneously and the athlete will have a painful swollen knee due to hemarthrosis and tenderness at the medial capsule. Lateral pressure on the patella while gently extending the knee will be met with obvious anxiety and resistance.

Management

If there is no obvious evidence of fracture, an attempted reduction of the dislocation can be made by first extending the knee. It can be helpful to massage the hamstring muscle and ask the athlete to relax it. As the patient allows more knee extension, exert gentle midline pressure directed to the lateral aspect of the patella. The patella should relocate in seconds to minutes. Difficulty with this maneuver suggests a fracture or displaced chondral fragment; the next step would be to splint the knee and refer to an emergency room for radiographs and reduction. Postreduction management follows the RICE protocol, with crutch use for those who can't bear weight. The leg should be elevated while the edema persists, with immediate quadriceps-strengthening exercises to prevent atrophy.

Neck Injuries

Injuries to the head and neck are the most frequent catastrophic sports injury. The four common school sports with the highest risk of head and spine injury are football, gymnastics, ice hockey, and wrestling. Nonschool sports risks far outweigh those from organized sports. Common causes of head injuries in this group are trampoline use, cycling, and snow sports.[10] Fortunately, many neck injuries are minimal strains, diagnosed after a quick history and physical examination. Axial loading is the most common mechanism for serious neck injury. Classic examples include the football player "spearing" or tackling head first, and the hockey player sliding head first into the boards. Axial loading can produce spinal fracture, dislocation, and quadriplegia at very low impact velocities—lower than for skull fractures. Extension spinal injuries are more serious than flexion injuries. With extension spine injury (whiplash), the anterior elements are disrupted and the posterior elements are compressed. In flexion injury, the anterior elements are compressed, causing anterior vertebral body fracture, chip fracture, and occasionally anterior dislocation.

Diagnosis

When an athlete is unconscious and motionless, an initial assessment is mandatory. Athletes with focal neurological deficits or marked neck pain should be suspected of having cervical spine injury until cleared by x-ray examination.

Management

The ABC (airway, breathing, and circulation) of emergency care apply, along with neck stabilization and initiation of emergency transport. Cervical spine injury is assumed until proven otherwise. Proper stabilization precautions must be carried out while the athlete is removed from the playing field or injury site. If the athlete is wearing a helmet, it should not be removed until arrival in the emergency room.

Closed Head Injuries

The definition of concussion by the Neurosurgical Committee on Head Injuries is "a clinical syndrome characterized by immediate and transient posttraumatic impairment of neural function, such as the alteration of consciousness disturbance of vision, equilibrium, etc., due to brainstem involvement."[11] There is also a complication of concussion called a " second-impact syndrome" in which fatal intracerebral edema is precipitated by a second blow to the head of an athlete who has persisting symptoms from an earlier concussion.[12] Fortunately, this syndrome is rare. If athletes have any persisting symptoms from any degree of concussion, they should not be allowed to play. Postconcussion syndrome consists of headache (especially with exertion), labyrinthine disturbance, fatigue, irritability, and impaired memory and concentration. These symptoms can persist for weeks or even months. Both football and snowboarding are common sports associated with closed head injuries.

Epidural hematoma results when the middle meningeal artery, which is embedded in a bony groove in the skull, tears as a result of a skull fracture, crossing this groove. Because the bleeding in this instance is arterial, accumulation of clot continues under high pressure and, as a result, serious brain injury can occur. Subdural hematomas are caused by the shearing forces applied to the bridging arachnoid veins that surround the brain.

Diagnosis

Reviewing the recognition and classification of concussion can simplify its management (Table 10.2). The classic description of an epidural hematoma is that of loss of consciousness in a variable period, followed by recovery of consciousness after which the patient is lucid. This is followed by the onset of increasingly severe headache; decreased level of consciousness; dilation of one pupil, usually on the same side as the clot; and decerebrate posturing and weakness, usually on the side opposite the hematoma. Patients with acute subdural hematoma are more likely to have a prolonged lucid interval following their injury and are less likely to be unconscious at admission than patients with epidural hematomas.

Management

Patients with closed head injuries need a thorough neurological evaluation, usually including a computed axial tomography (CAT) scan or magnetic resonance imaging (MRI). Return to competition should be

Table 10.2. **Grading of Head Injuries and Management**

Grade of concussion	Symptoms	Management
1	Brief confusion, <30 min, no LOC	No head imaging required unless focal deficit appears or LOC develops; may return to activity with head protection in 7 days
2	Prolonged amnesia or confusion, >30 min, no LOC	No head imaging required unless focal deficit appears or LOC develops; may return to activity with head protection in 21 days
3a	LOC <5 min; amnesia, confusion common	Computed tomography or magnetic resonance imaging recommended to rule out hemorrhage; no further sports activity with risk of head injury for remainder of season; helmet use in the future is strongly recommended
3b	LOC ≥5 min	

LOC = loss of consciousness.

deferred until all symptoms have abated and the guidelines described in Table 10.2 have been followed. Adequate head protection in skiers, snowboarders, and football players is an appropriate prevention measure and should be mandatory if the patient has a history of a previous concussion.

Shoulder Dislocation

Shoulder dislocation may occur when sufficient impact tears the anterior joint capsule of the glenohumeral joint, resulting in a slippage of the humeral head out of the glenoid fossa. In anterior glenohumeral dislocation there are two mechanisms of injury: a fall onto an outstretched hand, or a collision with a player or object with the shoulder abducted to 90 degrees and externally rotated. While the shoulder may dislocate posteriorly, an anterior–inferior dislocation is the most common. Careful examination to rule out humeral neck fracture is important before reduction of the shoulder in the field. Small avulsion fractures can occur at the attachment of the supraspinatus tendon (Fig. 10.3), but this injury will not preclude immediate reduction of the shoulder.

Diagnosis

Athletes who have anterior shoulder dislocation will often state that the shoulder has "popped out" and complain of excruciating pain. The athlete is unable to rotate the arm and has a hollow region just inferior to the acromion with an anterior bulge caused by the forward displacement of the humeral head. Subluxation of the shoulder may occur when the humerus slips out of the glenohumeral socket and then spontaneously relocates. Posterior subluxations are seen more commonly in athletes who use repetitive overhand motion such as swimmers and baseball and tennis players.

Management

Anterior dislocation is the only shoulder injury that requires prompt manipulation. The Rockwood technique involves an assistant who applies a long, folded towel around the ipsilateral axilla, crossing the upper anterior/posterior chest. Gentle traction is applied while the physician applies in-line traction at 45 degrees abduction on the injured extremity. Traction is gradually increased over several minutes. Successful reduction will manifest as a "thunk" when the humerus relocates in the glenoid cavity. If started immediately, the dislocation

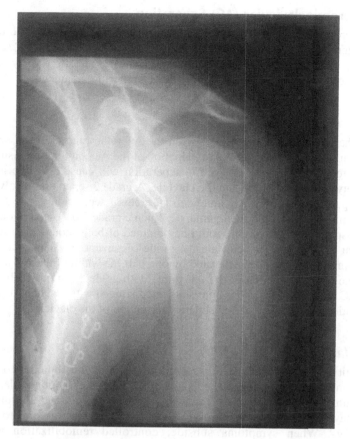

Fig. 10.3. Small avulsion fracture of the proximal humerus in a skier who sustained a shoulder dislocation.

should be reducible in 2 to 3 minutes. Postreduction radiographs are required. With the Stimson technique, the patient lies prone on a flat surface with the arm hanging down. A 5-pound weight is tied to the distal forearm. The reduction will usually take place within 20 minutes.[13] Scapular manipulation in a similar position has also been described as another method to relocate the shoulder with minimal traction.[13] If these attempts at early reduction are unsuccessful, reduction using analgesia or anesthesia can be attempted in the emergency room. In the patient who dislocates for the first time, the shoulder should be immobilized for 2 to 3 weeks. Rehabilitation may reduce the rate of recurrence with goals being the restoration of full shoulder abduction and strengthening of the rotator cuff muscles.[14]

Acromioclavicular (AC) Separation

Acromioclavicular separation may be caused by a direct blow to the lateral aspect of the shoulder or a fall on an outstretched arm. AC separations are classified as grades 1, 2, or 3 as determined by the involvement of the AC and/or the coracoclavicular ligaments.

Diagnosis

There will be discrete tenderness at the AC joint. In grade 1 AC separation, there is tenderness to palpation at the AC joint but no visible defect. Grade 2 or grade 3 AC separation will cause a visible gap between the acromion and the clavicle. A grade 2 separation involves a partial tear of the AC ligaments; a grade 3 separation is due to a complete tear of the AC ligaments. When a grade 2 or 3 separation is suspected, a radiograph should be obtained of both shoulders to rule out fracture and to delineate the grade of separation. With grade 2 injuries, the clavicle is elevated by one half the width of the AC joint due to the disruption of the AC joint. With grade 3 injuries both the AC and coracoclavicular ligaments are disrupted with resultant dislocation of the AC joint and superior migration of the clavicle.

Management

Initial management of AC separations requires the shoulder to be immobilized in a sling. The extent of medical intervention is determined by the grade of the injury. Those with grade 1 and 2 injuries may be treated conservatively with sling immobilization for 7 to 14 days. When symptoms subside, controlled remobilization and strengthening of the shoulder should begin. There is ongoing controversy regarding conservative versus operative management of the grade 3 injury. An orthopedic referral should be made for these athletes.

Brachial Plexus Injury

A brachial plexus injury, or "burner" or "stinger," is a temporary dysfunction of the neural structures in the brachial plexus after a blow to the head, neck, or shoulder. Burners are reported in football, wrestling, ice hockey, skiing, motocross, soccer, hiking, and equestrian sports.[15] Several mechanisms probably contribute to injuries to the brachial plexus, usually involving lateral flexion of the cervical spine with concomitant depression of one of the shoulders. Lateral flexion with rotation and extension of the cervical spine toward the symptomatic side causes a direct compression of the nerve roots, while lateral flexion with shoulder depression causes a traction injury to the nerves.[16]

Diagnosis

Typically the player experiences a sharp burning pain in the shoulder with paresthesia or dysesthesia radiating into the arm and hand. The patient may have associated sensory deficits, decreased reflexes, and weakness of the deltoid, biceps, supraspinatus, or infraspinatus muscles.

Management

If the neurological findings return to normal within a few minutes, the athlete may return to play. In 5% to 10% of patients, signs and symptoms will persist requiring referral to either a neurologist or a physiatrist.

Thumb and Finger Injuries

Extensor injuries of the distal phalangeal joints occur when there is avulsion of the extensor tendon from the distal phalanx with and without a fracture. This results in a "mallet "or "drop" finger. Proximal phalangeal joint injuries occur when there is avulsion of the central slip of the distal phalanx, resulting in a flexion "boutonniere" deformity. Metacarpophalangeal (MCP) joint sprain of the thumb ("gamekeeper's" thumb) is caused by a fall on an outstretched hand, causing forced abduction to the thumb.

Diagnosis

The distal or proximal phalanx is flexed and lacks active extension in extensor tendon ruptures. It is imperative that any distal interphalangeal (DIP) injury be evaluated for full extension to avoid missing a extensor tendon rupture. Gamekeeper's thumb causes pain and swelling over the ulnar aspect of the MCP joint and is made worse by abducting or extending the thumb. Complete tears of the ulnar collateral ligament are demonstrated by marked laxity in full extension.

Management

An x-ray should be obtained in all of the above injuries to rule out intraarticular fractures or avulsions that require orthopedic referral. In extensor tendon injuries, continued splinting of the distal finger joint in extension for at least 6 weeks is necessary. The treatment for a gamekeeper's thumb requires a thumb spica cast or splint protection for 4 to 6 weeks. During activity, the thumb can be protected by taping it to the index finger to prevent excessive abduction. A complete tear of the ulnar collateral ligament requires orthopedic referral for surgical repair.[17] Minor sprains can be rehabilitated in 3 to 4 weeks.

Specific Overuse Injuries

Shoulder Impingement Syndromes

Overuse injuries of the shoulder are most commonly seen in swimming, throwing, or racquet sports. Swimmers almost uniformly develop symptoms of this injury to varying degrees, especially those swimmers who regularly perform the butterfly stroke. Repetitive motions that abduct and retract the arm followed by antegrade (overhand) rotation of the glenohumeral joint can lead to impingement of the subacromial bursa and the supraspinatus tendon. Early in the course, only the subacromial bursa may be inflamed, but with progressive injury supraspinatus tendonitis develops and may become calcified. Other muscles that make up the rotator cuff can also be strained with this motion and eventually can lead to rotator cuff tears.

Diagnosis

Patients with impingement will complain of pain with abduction to varying degrees and especially with attempts to raise the arm above the level of the shoulder. The pain radiates deep from the subacromial space to the deltoid region and may be vague and not well localized. Palpation of the subacromial bursa under the coracoacromial ligament will often elicit pain deep to the acromion, as will internal rotation of the arm when abducted at 90 degrees with the elbow also flexed at 90 degrees. A second maneuver to detect impingement is to extend the arm forward so it is parallel to the ground and then internally rotate and abduct the arm across the chest while stabilizing the shoulder with the examiner's hand. Both maneuvers narrow the subacromial space to elicit symptoms. The "painful arc"—pain only within a limited range of abduction—may indicate an advanced calcific tendonitis of the supraspinatus tendon. Radiographic imaging may be useful if this finding is present, as calcific tendonitis may require more invasive treatment.

Management

Modification of shoulder activity and antiinflammatory measures [the RICE protocol, nonsteroidal antiinflammatory drugs (NSAIDs)] are instituted early. Swimmers will need to alter the strokes during their training periods and reduce the distance that they swim to the point that the pain is decreasing daily. Rehabilitation exercises should consist of both aggressive shoulder stretching to lengthen the coracoacromial ligament and improve range of motion. The use of an upper arm counterforce brace will alter the fulcrum of the biceps in such a way as to depress the humeral head further. Strength training of the supraspinatus and biceps internal and external rotator muscles should be performed to aid in depressing the humeral head when stressed, thus increasing the subacromial space. In advanced calcific tendonitis, steroid injection into the subacromial bursa or surgical removal of the calcific tendon may be required.[18]

Tennis Elbow (Lateral Epicondylitis)

Lateral epicondylitis is characterized by point tenderness of the lateral epicondyle at the attachment of the extensor carpi radialis brevis. The most common sports that cause this syndrome are tennis, racquetball, and cross-country skiing.[19] The mechanism of injury in all of the sports is the repetitive extension of the wrist against resistance. Adolescent or preadolescent athletes are at highest risk of significant injury if the growth plate that underlies the lateral epicondyle is not yet closed. If the inflammation of the epicondyle is not arrested, the soft growth cartilage can fracture and rotate the bony attachment of the extensor ligaments, requiring surgical reimplantation of the epicondyle. Without surgery, a permanent deformity of the elbow will result.

Diagnosis

Patients will complain of pain with active extension of the wrist localized to the upper forearm and lateral epicondyle. There is usually marked tenderness of the epicondyle itself. Pain with grasping a weighted cup (Canard's test) or with resisted dorsiflexion is also diagnostic. X-ray studies are not necessary but may show calcific changes to the extensor aponeurosis in chronic cases. Comparison views of the unaffected elbow may be helpful in the adolescent in whom a stress fracture is suspected and the growth plate is not yet closed. Stress fractures of the lateral epicondyle are best diagnosed with a technetium-99 (Te-99) bone scan.

Management

Rest, NSAIDs, and ice to the area are the initial treatment modalities. Modification of the gripped object (racquet or ski pole) with a thicker grip will reduce the stress on the extensors. A counterforce brace worn over the belly of the forearm extensors or a volar cock-up splint can be used to relieve symptoms and alter the dynamic fulcrum of the muscles. Steroid injections superficial to the aponeurosis can be used in more refractory cases but should be limited to three injections.[20] Steroids should not be used in patients who may have a stress fracture or if the growth plates have not yet closed. Gradual return to the sport may begin immediately in grade 1 or 2 injuries, or as soon as the tenderness has resolved in higher grade injuries.

Lumbar Spondylolysis/Spondylolisthesis

Spondylolysis (fracture of the pars interarticularis) of the vertebrae results from repeated forced hyperextension of the spine. Spondylolisthesis (slippage of one vertebrae over another) may result from the facet joint degeneration induced by spondylolysis. Young preadolescent gymnasts are at highest risk for developing spondylolysis but it can also be seen in weight lifters, runners, swimmers who perform the butterfly stroke, divers, and football players.[21] In one large study, up to 10% of adolescent female gymnasts had spondylolysis.[22] Spondylolisthesis usually occurs in older teens and develops primarily at the L5-S1 joint. Their prognosis is worse than those with isolated spondylolysis.

Diagnosis

The athlete usually complains of unilateral back pain that worsens with rotation of the trunk. There is usually regional spasm of the paraspinous musculature and the hamstrings. Pain from spondylolisthesis may cause radicular symptoms in the L5-S1 distribution. Lateral and anteroposterior (AP) x-rays of the spine may not reveal pars interarticularis pathology so oblique films should be added. Even if the x-rays are normal, if the diagnosis is suspected, restriction of the activity is necessary until repeat films are done in 4 to 6 weeks. A Te-99 bone scan is a sensitive test for detecting pars interarticularis fractures or stress reactions.

Management

Rest is essential in both of these conditions. Bone scans can be used to follow the healing process but costs may be prohibitive. Resolution of symptoms is an adequate indicator of healing. The athlete may continue to train in sports that do not result in hyperextension or rotation of the spine (e.g., cycling, stair-climbing) as long as the back symptoms are improving. Referral to a physical therapist for neutral spine stability exercises is warranted.

Low-grade spondylolisthesis can be managed conservatively by restriction of activity until the pain has resolved. Serial x-rays every 4 to 6 months can monitor progression in athletes who returned to their sport after the symptoms resolved. High-grade spondylolisthesis (>25% displacement of the vertebral body) can also be managed conservatively, but the patient must be permanently restricted from contact or collision sports. Bracing or surgical repair of spondylolisthesis may be required if pain is severe or persistent nerve root irritation is present.[23]

Retropatellar (Patellofemoral) Pain Syndrome

Retropatellar pain syndrome (RPPS) is most commonly found in patients participating in running, hiking, or cycling. The symptoms probably represent the majority of knee pain complaints in athletes. Retropatellar pain is caused by the repetitive glide of the patella over the femoral condyles, which can lead to inflammation of the retropatellar synovium or the cartilage itself. The glide of the patella is usually laterally displaced in athletes who have recurrent symptoms. Factors that increase this friction are instability of the knee from previous injury, valgus deformity of the knee, deficient vastus medialis obliquus muscle strength, patella alta, or recent increase in running program. Relative valgus stress on the knee is created in patients with abnormal Q angles, pes planus, femoral anteversion, or external tibial torsion causing lateral displacement of the patella. If progressive, RPPS can progress to chondromalacia patellae with destruction of the retropatellar cartilage.

Diagnosis

Patients with RPPS present with vague retropatellar or peripatellar pain, which is usually most significant several hours after exercise. Walking downhill or downstairs, bending at the knees, and kneeling exacerbate pain symptoms. In more advanced cases, pain can be constant, occurring during and after exercise. Oddly, patients often experience pain if the knee is not moved enough; i.e., if left flexed for several minutes, pain will develop. The examination of the knee should first include inspection of the patient's entire leg, feet, and hips to assess for a significant Q angle, torsional deformities, leg length discrepancy, or pes planus. On palpation of the knee, the lateral posterior margins of the patella should be palpated with the patella deviated laterally to detect tenderness of the retropatellar surface. This should also be repeated on the medial aspect of the patella with medial deviation. Effusions are usually absent in RPPS. A compression test of the patella is performed with the patient relaxing and then flexing the quadriceps group while the patella is displaced distally by the examiner. Fine crepitus with this test may indicate synovial inflammation but it is not specific. Coarse crepitus or popping with significant pain is indicative of chondromalacia. Sunrise views of the knees may reveal radiographic evidence of retropatellar degeneration, but usually these findings are present only in advanced cases and are not necessary for diagnosis.[24]

Management

For athletes with symptoms only at higher training levels, reduction of the exacerbating activity and NSAID use are the first steps. If the patient has a grade 3 or 4 injury, then cessation of the exacerbating activity for 2 to 4 weeks until the pain is no longer present at rest is necessary. Selective strengthening of the vastus medialis obliquus (VMO), orthotics, and alteration of mechanical forces when pedaling (for cyclists) can also relieve symptoms. Lateral deviation of the foot while extending the knee allows more medial tracking of the patella during exercise and forces the VMO to perform more of the quadriceps function. Stretching to reduce both hamstring and quadriceps tension is an important component of the rehabilitation of RPPS. As with all overuse injuries, a graduated increase in exercise duration at a rate of 10% per week, with relative rest periods every 3 to 4 weeks, may prevent recurrence of the symptoms.

Tibial Periostitis ("Shin Splints")

Tibial periostitis is the most common overuse injury in recreational runners and is often confused with other lower leg pain syndromes.[25] Any pain in the tibial area is often labeled "shin splints" but must be differentiated from anterior compartment syndrome, patellar tendonitis, or a simple muscular strain. The primary cause of tibial periostitis is mechanical; the attachment of a calf muscle is strained due to the pounding of running on a mechanically deficient foot. A recent increase in duration of running often triggers shin splints if the increase is too rapid and there is no rest phase. Over 4 to 8 weeks after such increases in training, this condition progresses to involve the bone by disrupting the periosteum and cortex.

Diagnosis

Most patients with this syndrome have pes planus, which results in tibialis posterior tendonitis initially. Their pain is localized to the lower third of the medial aspect of the tibia. Patients with pes cavus have anterior tibialis tendonitis with pain localized laterally on the middle or upper tibia. If other calf flexors are involved, the pain may be deep in the calf, resembling a deep vein thrombosis (DVT). Homans' sign may be positive in these patients because the posterior aspect of the tibia is inflamed. If point tenderness is present, x-ray studies are indicated, with careful attention being paid to subtle changes in the cortical margin in the area of pain.

Management

Table 10.3 delineates rehabilitation strategies for this injury. The importance of adequate rest and graduated resumption of exercise with cycled rest phases cannot be overemphasized.[26] Aggressive stretching of the calf muscles, twice daily icing the affected area, and NSAIDs are essential adjuncts to adjustments in the training program. Corrective arch supports for either pes planus or pes cavus are necessary if these conditions are present. Combining strength training with resumption of running will enhance tendon healing and adaptive cortical thickening.

Jones' Fractures (Proximal Fifth Metatarsal Fractures)

Overuse injuries of the foot can occur in multiple sites including the metatarsal, tarsal, and sesamoid bones. Jones' and sesamoid bone fractures have very high rates of nonunion (50–90%).[27] These stress fractures must be detected and treated early to prevent this complication. Jones' fractures are primarily seen in distance runners, especially in those with a recent increase in activity. There is usually a history of antecedent pain for several weeks at the attachment of the peroneus brevis tendon to the proximal fifth metatarsal.

Diagnosis

Pain and tenderness at the site are universal. Inversion of the ankle, causing stress of the peroneus brevis tendon, or attempts to evert the

Table 10.3. **Overuse Injuries: Staging and Rehabilitation**

Stage	Symptoms	Rehabilitation
1	Pain with maximal exertion, resolves after event; nonfocal exam	Decrease activity to 50–70%, ice, NSAIDs for 7 days; every other day training
2	Pain with minimal exertion, resolves in <24 hours; minimal tenderness	Decrease activity to 50%, ice, NSAIDs for 10–14 days; every other day training
3	Pain despite rest, not resolved within 48 hours; tender on exam, mild swelling of tendon	Stop activity 2–4 weeks or until pain free; ice, NSAIDs; resume training at 50%, increase by 10% per week; every 4 weeks reduce to 50%
4	Continual pain, stress fracture, point tenderness, and swelling	Immobilize if indicated; rest 4–6 weeks until pain free; ice, NSAIDs; resume training at 50%, increase by 10% per week; every 4 weeks reduce to 50%

NSAID = nonsteroidal antiinflammatory drug.

foot against stress also localize pain to the proximal head of the fifth metatarsal. Radiographs may show evidence of cortical thickening, sclerotic changes within the medullary bone, or a true fracture line. The more proximal the fracture, the higher the risk of delayed union. If the radiographs are negative, but if there is significant tenderness, then a bone scan should be performed because of the high rate of false-negative radiographs for this fracture.

Management

All athletes with evidence of stress fracture on bone scan or sclerotic changes on x-ray should be referred for possible screw placement.[28] If there is evidence only of a periosteal reaction, without visible fracture or medullary sclerosis, the foot should be placed in a non weight-bearing short leg cast for 4 to 6 weeks and follow-up films obtained when pain free to ensure that healing has been complete. Despite appropriate care, avascular necrosis may occur, requiring grafting of the bone. After the fracture is healed, the athlete may gradually return to the activity, with close follow-up to prevent recurrence of symptoms.[29]

Prevention of Injuries

The primary focus of injury prevention stems from understanding the mechanisms of injury. In contact or collision sports, appropriate protective equipment is essential in reducing the severity of injuries sustained by the participants. Wearing protective helmets substantially reduces risk of head injuries in many collision sports. In sports where the risk of falls is prominent, use of wrist guards and knee pads can reduce injuries to these joints. Alpine skiers must use releasable bindings that are adjusted appropriately for their weight and skill level to reduce the risk of ligamentous knee injuries. Overuse injuries can be prevented by developing graded training programs that allow time for compensatory changes in tendons and bones to prevent inflammation. Orthotics and focused training of muscle groups can correct mechanical problems that could lead to overuse injuries.

The second aspect of injury prevention is maximizing the strength, proprioceptive skills, and the flexibility of the athlete. Appropriate off-season and preseason training of athletes, coaches, and trainers can substantially reduce injuries during the regular season.

References

1. Cook PC, Leit ME. Issues in the pediatric athlete. Orthop Clin North Am 1995;26:453–64.
2. Patel DR. Sports injuries in adolescents. Med Clin North Am 2000;84:983–1007.
3. Brody DM. Running injuries. Clin Sym 1987;39:23–5.
4. Hulkko A, Orava S. Stress fractures in athletes. Int J Sports Med 1987; 8:221–6.
5. Clanton TO, Porter DA Primary care of foot and ankle injuries in the athlete. Clin Sports Med 1997;16:435–66.
6. Brostrom L. Sprained ankles, I. Anatomic lesions in recent sprains. Acta Chir Scand 1964;128:483–95.
7. Stiell IG. Decision rules for the use of radiography in acute ankle injuries. JAMA 1993;269:1127–32.
8. Perlman M, Leveille D, DeLeonibus J, et al. Inversion lateral ankle trauma: differential diagnosis, review of the literature and prospective study. J Foot Surg 1987;26:95–135.
9. Dyment PG. Athletic injuries. Pediatr Rev 1989;10(10):1–13.
10. Proctor MR, Cantu RC. Head and spine injuries in young athletes. Clin Sports Med 2000;19:693–715.
11. Committee on Head Injury Nomenclature of the Congress of Neurological Surgeons. Glossary of head injury including some definitions of injury to the cervical spine. Clin Neurosurg 1966;12:386.
12. Cantu RC. Second impact syndrome. Physician Sports Med 1992;20: 55–66.
13. Hergengroeder AC. Acute shoulder, knee and ankle injuries. Part 1: diagnosis and management. Adolesc Health Update 1996;8(2):1–8.
14. Blake R, Hoffman J. Emergency department evaluation and treatment of the shoulder and humerus. Emerg Med Clin North Am 1999;17:859–76.
15. Aronen JC, Regan K. Decreasing the incidence of recurrence of first time anterior shoulder dislocations with rehabilitation. Am J Sports Med 1984;12:283–91.
16. Archambault JL. Brachial plexus stretch injury. J Am Coll. Health 1983; 31(6):256–60.
17. Vereschagin KS, Weins JJ, Fanton GS, Dillingham MF. Burners, don't overlook or underestimate them. Phys Sportsmed 1991;19(9):96–106.
18. Kahler DM, McLue FC. Metacarpophalangeal and proximal interphalangeal joint injuries of the hand, including the thumb. Clin Sports Med 1992;11:5–76.
19. Smith DL, Campbell SM. Painful shoulder syndromes: diagnosis and management. J Gen Intern Med 1992;7:328–39.
20. Safran MR. Elbow injuries in athletes: a review. Clin Orthop 1995;310: 257–77.
21. Mehlhoff TL, Bennett B. The elbow. In: Mellion MB, Walsh WM, Shelton GL, eds. The team physician handbook. Philadelphia: Hanley & Belfus, 1990. p. 334–345.
22. Wilhite J, Huurman WW. The thoracic and lumbar spine. In: Mellion MB, Walsh WM, Shelton GL, eds. The team physician handbook. Philadelphia: Hanley & Belfus, 1990. p. 374–400.

23. Jackson DW, Wiltse LL. Low back pain in young athletes. Phys Sportsmed 1974;2:53–60.
24. Smith JA, Hu SS. Disorders of the pediatric and adolescent spine. Orthop Clin North Am 1999;30:487–99.
25. Davidson K. Patellofemoral pain syndrome. Am Fam Physician 1993;48:1254–62.
26. Batt ME. Shin splints—a review of terminology. Clin J Sports Med 1995;5:53–7.
27. Stanitski CL. Common injuries in preadolescent and adolescent athletes. Sports Med 1989;7:32–41.
28. Orava S, Hulkko A. Delayed unions and nonunions of stress fractures in athletes. Am J Sports Med 1988;16:378–82.
29. Lawrence SJ, Bolte MJ. Jones fractures and related fractures of the fifth metatarsal. Foot Ankle 1993;14:358–65.

11
Care of Acute Lacerations

Bryan J. Campbell and
Douglas J. Campbell

The optimum management of lacerations requires knowledge of skin anatomy and the physiology of wound healing. Such knowledge facilitates proper management of wounds of varying depth and complexity. By understanding the healing process, the family physician can maximize the options for repair and minimize the dangers of dehiscence and infection. The goals of primary closure are to stop bleeding, prevent infection, preserve function, and restore appearance. The patient always benefits from a physician who treats the patient gently, handles the tissue carefully, understands anatomy, and appreciates the healing process.[1,2]

Skin Anatomy

Figure 11.1 represents a model of the skin and the underlying tissue down to structures such as bone or muscle. Two additional features of skin anatomy that affect the repair of injuries are cleavage lines and wrinkles. Lines of cleavage are also known as Langer's lines. These lines are formed by the collagen bundles that lie parallel in the dermis. An incision or repair along these lines lessens disruption of collagen bundles and decreases new collagen formation and therefore causes less scarring. Wrinkle lines are not always consistent with Langer's lines. If a laceration is not in an area of apparent

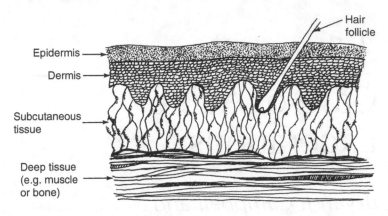

Fig. 11.1. Model of skin and subcutaneous tissue.

wrinkling, following the basic outline of Langer's lines results in the best repair.

Wound Healing

Phase One: Inflammatory Phase

The substrate, or inflammatory, phase occurs during the first 5 to 6 days after injury. Leukocytes, histamines, prostaglandins, and fibrinogen, delivered to the injury site via blood and lymphatic channels, attempt to neutralize bacteria and foreign material. The amount of inflammation present in a wound is related to the presence of necrotic tissue, which is increased by dead space and impaired circulation. Specific measures that reduce the inflammatory response include debridement, removal of foreign material, cleaning, control of bleeding, and precise tissue coaptation.

Phase Two: Fibroblastic Phase

The fibroblastic, or collagen, phase occupies days 6 though 20 after injury. Fibroblasts enter the wound rapidly and begin collagen synthesis, which binds the wound together. As the collagen content rises, the wound strength increases until the supporting ligature can be removed. Compromise of the vascular supply can inhibit the development of collagen synthesis and interfere with healing.

Phase Three: Maturation (Remodeling) Phase

The wound continues to undergo remodeling for 18 to 24 months, during which time collagen synthesis continues and retraction occurs. Normally during this time the scar becomes softer and less conspicuous. The prominent color of the scar gradually fades, resulting in a hue consistent with the surrounding skin. Aberrations of the maturation process can result in an unsightly scar such as a keloid. Such scars are due to a combination of inherited tendencies and extrinsic factors of the wound. Proper technique in wound care and repair minimizes the extrinsic contribution to keloid formation. If it is necessary to revise an unsightly scar, the ideal delay is 18 months or more after the initial repair.

Anesthesia

Under most circumstances it is preferable to anesthetize the wound prior to preparation for closure. Before applying anesthesia, the wound is inspected using a slow, gentle, aseptic technique to ascertain the extent of injury including an assessment of the neurovascular supply. At this time a decision is made to refer the patient if the complexity of the wound warrants consultation.

Topical Agents

When appropriate, topical anesthesia is ideal, as pain can be relieved without causing more discomfort or anxiety. Small lacerations may be closed without additional medications.

PAC (Pontocaine/Adrenaline/Cocaine) and TAC (Tetracaine/Adrenaline/Cocaine)

Pontocaine or tetracaine 2%/aqueous epinephrine (adrenaline) 1:1000/cocaine (PAC) is the most commonly used topical agent.[3,4] It may be prepared in a 100-mL volume by mixing 25 mL of 2% tetracaine, 50 mL of 1:1000 aqueous epinephrine, 11.8 g of cocaine, and sterile normal saline to a volume of 100 mL.

Placing a saturated pledget over the wound for 5 to 15 minutes often provides adequate local anesthesia. Blanching of the skin beyond the margin of the wound allows an estimation of adequate anesthesia. Further anesthesia may be applied by injection if necessary.

Emla

Emla is a commercially available preparation of 2.5% lidocaine/ 2.5% prilocaine in a buffered vehicle. It is squeezed onto the skin surface and covered with an occlusive dressing. Its efficacy is similar to that of TAC, but it takes nearly twice as long to anesthetize the skin (30 minutes). The same guideline of skin blanching applies to the use of Emla.

Ethyl Chloride

A highly volatile fluid, ethyl chloride comes in commercially prepared glass bottles with a sprayer lid. This fluid can be sprayed onto the skin surface by inverting the bottle and pressing the lid. The flammable fluid chills the skin rapidly. The agent may be applied until skin frosting occurs. It provides brief anesthesia, allowing immediate placement of a needle without causing additional pain.

Injectable Agents

Lidocaine

Lidocaine produces moderate duration of anesthesia (about 1–2 hours) when used in a 1% or 2% solution. When mixed with 1:100,000 aqueous epinephrine, the anesthetic effect is prolonged (2–6 hours), and there is a local vasoconstrictive effect. Any anesthetic mixed with epinephrine should be used with caution on fingers, toes, ears, nose, or the penis to avoid risk of ischemia and subsequent necrosis. Occasional toxicity occurs with lidocaine, but most reactions are due to inadvertent intravascular injection. Manifestations of toxicity include tinnitus, numbness, confusion, and rarely progression to coma. True allergic reactions are unusual.

It is possible to reduce the discomfort of lidocaine injection by buffering the solution with the addition of sterile sodium bicarbonate.[5–8] A solution of 9 mL of lidocaine plus 1 mL of sodium bicarbonate (44 mEq/50 mL) is less painful to inject but provides the same level of anesthesia as the unbuffered solution. It is also possible to buffer other injectable agents including those with epinephrine. However, epinephrine is unstable at a pH above 5.5 and is commercially prepared in solutions below that pH. Therefore, any buffered local anesthetic with epinephrine must be used within a short time of preparation.[9] Warming a buffered solution to body temperature provides additional reduction of the pain of injection. Buffering also appears to increase the antibacterial properties of anesthetic solutions.[10]

Additional Agents

Mepivacaine (Carbocaine) produces longer anesthesia than lidocaine (about 45–90 minutes). It is not used with epinephrine. Reactions are similar to those seen with lidocaine. Procaine (Novocain) works quickly but has a short duration (usually less than 30–45 minutes). It has a wide safety margin and may be used with epinephrine. Bupivacaine (Marcaine) is the longest-acting local anesthetic (approximately 6–8 hours). It is often used for nerve blocks or may be mixed with lidocaine for problems that take longer to repair. It is also useful for injecting into a wound to provide postprocedural pain relief. It may be mixed with epinephrine and is available in 0.25%, 0.50%, and 0.75% solutions.

Diphenhydramine

Diphenhydramine (Benadryl) may also be used as an injectable anesthetic.[11] It is somewhat more painful to inject than lidocaine but has an efficacy similar to that of lidocaine. Diphenhydramine may be prepared in a 0.5% solution by mixing a 1-mL vial of 50 mg diphenhydramine with 9 mL of saline. This solution is useful when a patient claims an allergy to all injectable anesthetics.

Anesthetic Methods

Infiltration Blocks

Infiltration blocks are useful for most laceration repairs. The wound is infiltrated by multiple injections into the skin and subcutaneous tissue. Using a long needle and a fan technique decreases the number of injection sites and therefore decreases the pain to the patient. Using a 27-gauge or smaller needle to inject through the open wound margin also minimizes the patient's discomfort, as does moving from an anesthetized area slowly toward the unanesthetized tissue.

Field Blocks

Field blocks result in similar pain control but may distort the wound margin less and are useful where accurate wound approximation is necessary (e.g., the vermillion border). The area around the wound is injected in a series of wheals completely around the wound, thereby blocking the cutaneous nerve supply to the laceration. This technique is more time-consuming but produces longer-lasting anesthesia. Another option to reduce the initial pain of the injection is to produce a small wheal using buffered sterile water and then injecting the anesthetic through the wheal. The buffered water has a brief anesthetic action.

Nerve Blocks

Nerve blocks are most commonly effected by injecting a nerve proximal to the injury site. The most frequent use of this technique is the digital block performed by injecting anesthetic into the webbing between the digits at the metacarpophalangeal joint on each side of the digit (Fig. 11.2). Mouth and tongue lacerations are repairable using dental blocks. It is useful to receive practical instruction in such blocks from a dental colleague.

Sedation

The Task Force on Sedation and Analgesia by Non Anesthesiologists[12] provides excellent protocols for sedative use by family physicians. Under adequate observation sedative agents can help the doctor deal

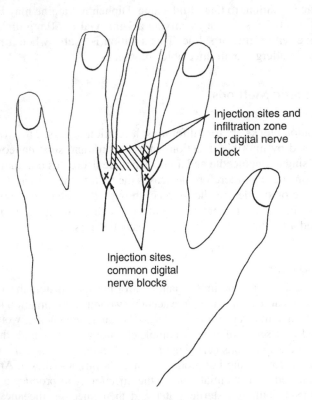

Injection sites and infiltration zone for digital nerve block

Injection sites, common digital nerve blocks

Fig. 11.2. Digital nerve block.

with difficult patients. For all agents described herein, it is imperative that there be appropriate monitoring and that adequate resuscitation equipment be readily available. The welfare of the patient is of prime concern, and such medications should not be used solely for the provider's convenience.

Ketamine

Ketamine is a phencyclidine derivative. It provides a dissociative state resulting in a trancelike condition and may provide amnesia for the procedure. Ketamine can be administered by many routes, but the most practical for laceration repair is the oral method. It usually results in significant analgesia without hypotension, decreased heart rate, or decreased respiratory drive. The use of proper monitoring and the availability of resuscitation equipment is mandatory. Oral ketamine can be prepared by adding 2.5 mL of ketamine hydrochloride injection (100 mg/mL) to 7.5 mL of flavored syrup. It is then given at a dose of 10 mg/kg. Sedation occurs over 20 to 45 minutes after ingestion. The most common side effects include nystagmus, random extremity movements, and vomiting during the recovery stage.[13]

Midazolam (Versed)

Midazolam is a benzodiazepine with typical class effects of hypnosis, amnesia, and anxiety reduction. It is readily absorbed and has a short elimination half-life. It may be given as a single dose via the nasal, oral, rectal, or parenteral route. The rectal route is useful when the patient is combative. A cooperative patient prefers oral or nasal administration (oral dose 0.5 mg/kg; nasal dose 0.25 mg/kg, by nasal drops). Injectable midazolam is used to make a solution that may be given orally or nasally. The drug should be made into a 5 mg/mL solution. For oral use it may be added to punch or apple juice to improve the taste. The maximum dose for children by any route is 8 mg.

For rectal administration, a 6-French (F) feeding tube is attached to an angiocath connected to a 5-mL syringe. The lubricated catheter is then inserted into the rectum and the drug injected followed by a syringe full of air to propel the medication into the rectum. The tube is then withdrawn and the patient's buttocks are held together for approximately 1 minute. The dose is 0.45 mg/kg by this route. The medication may begin to work as soon as 10 minutes after administration. Side effects may be delayed, so the patient should be observed for at least an hour as the duration of a single dose lasts about an hour. Some burning can occur when the nasal route is used. Inconsolable agitation may appear regardless of the route of administration. This side effect of agitated crying resolves after several hours. Vomiting may also occur.[12,14,15]

Fentanyl

Fentanyl is a powerful synthetic opioid that produces rapid, short-lasting sedation and analgesia. Like other opioids, its effects are reversible, and it has limited cardiovascular effects. Although it can be given in many forms, oral transmucosal fentanyl citrate (OTFC) is available commercially in a lollipop (Fentanyl Oralet). This drug, commonly used as an preanesthetic medication, is available in three dosage forms (200, 300, and 400 mg). The dose for adults is 5 mg/kg to a maximum of 400 mg regardless of weight. Pediatric dosages begin at 5 mg/kg to a maximum of 15 mg/kg or 400 mg (whichever is less). Children weighing less than 15 kg should not receive fentanyl. OTFC effects are apparent 5 to 10 minutes after sucking the Oralet. The maximum effect is usually achieved about 30 minutes after use, but effects may persist for several hours. Side effects are common but usually minor. About half of patients develop transient pruritus, 15% notice dizziness, and at least one third develop vomiting. The most dangerous effect is hypoventilation, which can be fatal.[12,16,17] Oversedation or respiratory depression responds to naloxone.

Nitrous Oxide

Nitrous oxide is a rapid-acting anesthetic that works within 3 to 5 minutes with a similar duration after cessation of administration.[18] Commercial equipment is available to deliver a mixture of nitrous oxide and oxygen at various ratios (usually 30–50% N_2O/50–70% O_2). Side effects include nausea in about 10% to 15% of patients with occasional emesis. The efficacy of nitrous oxide is known to be variable. Although some patients object to the use of the mask, many patients prefer using a specially designed self-administration mask. Nitrous oxide can cause expansion of gas-filled body pockets, and for that reason it should not be used in patients with head injuries, pneumothoraces, bowel obstructions, or middle ear effusions.

Wound Preparation

Proper preparation of a wound can improve the success of aesthetically acceptable healing. The wound should be closed as soon as possible, although most lacerations heal well if closed within 24 hours after the injury. After anesthesia, proper cleansing should be accomplished by wiping, scrubbing, and irrigating with normal saline using a large syringe with or without a 22-gauge needle, which produces enough velocity to clean most wounds. Antiseptic soaps such as hexachlorophene (pHisoHex), chlorhexidine gluconate (Hibiclens), or povidone-iodine (Betadine) can also be used, but one should be aware that all of these cleansing agents with the exception of normal saline will delay wound healing to some extent by destroying fibroblasts and leukocytes as well as bacteria. Sterile scrub brushes may be useful for cleaning grossly contaminated lesions.

After washing and irrigation, the area is draped with sterile towels to create a clean field. The wound is then explored using sterile technique to confirm the depth of injury, ascertain whether injury to underlying tissue has occurred, rule out the presence of any foreign body, and determine the adequacy of anesthesia. After examination, debridement is performed if necessary.

Debridement is the process of converting an irregular dirty wound to a clean one with smooth edges. Wound margins that are crushed, mangled, or devitalized are excised unless it is unwise to do so. Tissue in areas such as the lip or eyelid should be removed with extreme caution. It is pointless to increase the deformity when a somewhat imperfect scar can provide a more functional result. If a considerable amount of tissue has been crushed, initial removal of all the damaged tissue may result in undesirable function (such as would occur if the skin over a joint were removed). Such injuries should be closed loosely using subcutaneous absorbable sutures. The scar can be revised later if necessary.

The initial incision is made with a scalpel followed by excision with a pair of sharp tissue scissors. The edges should be perpendicular to the skin surface or even slightly undercut to facilitate eversion of the skin margins (Fig. 11.3). In hairy areas incisions should parallel the hair shafts to minimize the likelihood of hairless areas around the healed wound (Fig. 11.4).

After debridement the skin edges are held together to see if it is possible to approximate them with minimal tension. Generally, it is necessary to undermine the skin to achieve greater mobility of the surface by releasing some of the subcutaneous skin attachments that prevent the skin from sliding (Fig. 11.5). This step takes place in the subcutaneous layer and can be done with a scalpel or scissors. The wound is then undermined circumferentially about 4 to 5 mm from the edge of the margin. The undermining should be equal across the wound and widest where the skin needs to move the most, usually the center of the cut.

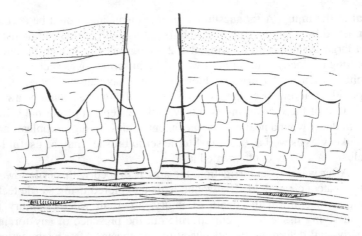

Fig. 11.3. Slight undercutting of the wound edges facilitates slight eversion of the wound edge.

Hemostasis can be accomplished most easily by simple pressure on the wound site for 5 to 10 minutes. If pressure is unsuccessful, bleeders may be carefully cauterized or ligated. Cautery or ligation can hinder healing if large amounts of tissue are damaged. Small vessels can be controlled with absorbable suture if necessary, but large arterial

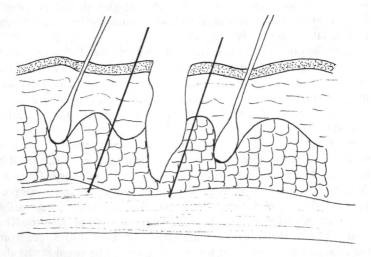

Fig. 11.4. Parallel debridement in a hairy area avoids damaging hair follicles.

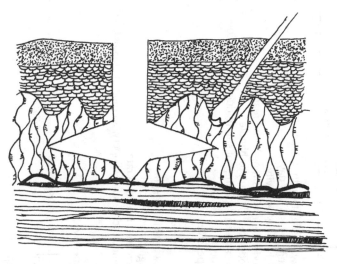

Fig. 11.5. Undermining the subdermal layer facilitates closure.

bleeders may need to be controlled with permanent ligature if it is possible to do so without compromising the distal circulation. If oozing persists, the wound is closed with a drain (e.g., a sterile rubber band or Penrose drain) left in the wound several days. An overlying pressure dressing minimizes bleeding. Advancing the drain every other day permits healing with minimal hematoma formation.

Wound Closure

Suture options are listed in Table 11.1. Absorbable materials are gradually broken down and absorbed by tissue; nonabsorbable sutures are made from chemicals that are encapsulated by the body and thus isolated from tissue. Monofilament sutures are less irritating to tissue but are more difficult to handle and require more knots than braided sutures. Stitches placed through the epidermis are done with nonabsorbable materials to minimize the tissue reactivity that occurs with absorbable stitches. Reverse cutting needles in a three-eighths or one-half circle design are available in various sizes for each type of suture.

A well-closed wound has three characteristics: the margins are approximated without tension, the tissue layers are accurately aligned, and dead space is eliminated. Deep stitches are placed in layers that hold the suture, such as the fat–fascial junction or the derma–fat

Table 11.1. **Common Suture Materials**

Suture	Advantages	Disadvantages
Absorbable		
Catgut	Inexpensive	Low tensile strength
		Strength lasts 4–5 days
		High tissue reactivity
Chromic catgut	Inexpensive	Moderate tensile strength and reactivity
Polyglycolic acid (Dexon)	Low tissue reactivity	Moderately difficult to handle
Polyglactic acid (Vicryl)	Easy handling	Occasional "spitting" of suture due to absorption delay
	Good tensile strength	
Polyglyconate (Maxon)	Easy handling	Expensive
	Good tensile strength	
Nonabsorbable		
Silk	Handles well	Low tensile strength
	Moderately inexpensive	High tissue reactivity
		Increased infection rate
Nylon (Ethilon, Dermilon)	High tensile strength	Difficult to handle; slippery; so many knots needed
	Minimal tissue reactivity	
	Inexpensive	
Polypropylene (Proline SurgiPro)	No tissue reaction	Expensive
	Stretches, accommodates swelling	
Braided polyester (Mersilene, Ethiflex)	Handles well	Tissue drag if uncoated
	Knots secure	Expensive
Polybutester (Novofil)	Elastic, accommodates swelling and retraction	Expensive

junction. A buried knot technique is the preferred method for placing deep sutures. Deep sutures provide most of the strength of the repair, and skin sutures approximate the skin margins and improve the cosmetic result (Fig. 11.6).

Suture Techniques[19–21]

Simple Interrupted Stitch

A simple interrupted stitch is placed by passing the needle through the skin surface at right angles, placing the suture   as wide as it is deep. The goal is to place sutures that slightly evert the edge of the wound (Fig. 11.7). This maneuver produces a slightly raised scar that recedes during the remodeling stage of healing and leaves a smooth scar. The opposite margin is approximated using a mirror image of the first placement. Following the natural radius of the curved needle places the suture in such a way as to evert the wound margin. It can be modified to correctly approximate the margins when the wound edges are asymmetric[1] (Fig. 11.8). Occasionally a wound exhibits excessively everted margins. By reversing the usual approach and taking a stitch that is wider at the top than at the base, the wound can be inverted,

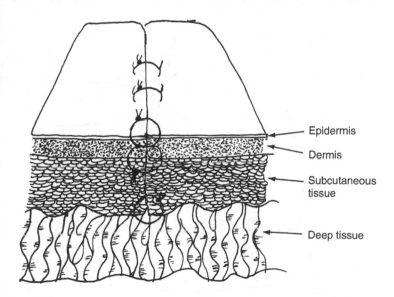

Fig. 11.6. Layer closure showing sutures in the epidermis, at the dermal–epidermal junction, and at the dermal–fat junction.

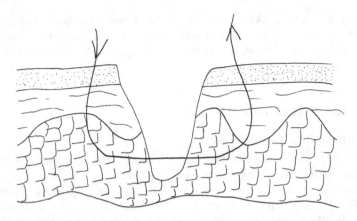

Fig. 11.7. Simple interrupted suture with placement to facilitate wound eversion.

improving the cosmetic appearance (Fig. 11.9). A useful general rule is that the entrance and exit points should be 2 mm from the margin for facial wounds but may be farther apart on other surfaces.[1,2] The open-loop knot (Fig. 11.10) avoids placing the suture under excessive tension and facilitates removal of the stitch. The first throw of the knot

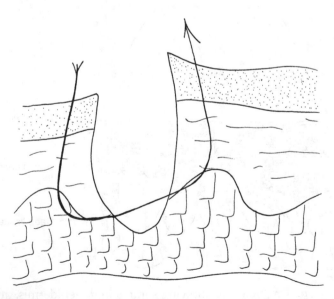

Fig. 11.8. Placement of suture in an asymmetric wound.

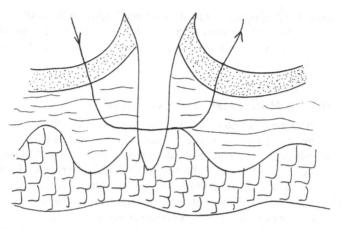

Fig. 11.9. Suture placement in a wound with everted edges.

with two loops ("surgeon's knot") is placed with just enough tension to approximate the wound margin. The second throw, a single loop, is tied, leaving a little space so no additional tension is placed on the first loop. Subsequent throws can be tightened snugly without increasing tension on the wound edge. Pulling all the knots to the same side of

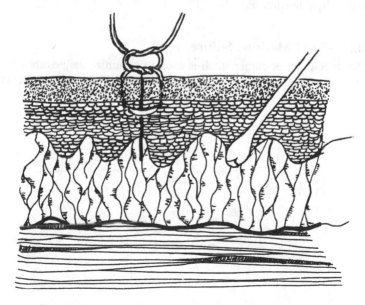

Fig. 11.10. Model of skin showing surgeon's knot.

the wound makes suture removal easier and improves the aesthetics of the repair. As a rule of thumb one should put at least the same number of knots of a monofilament suture as the size of the ligature (e.g., five knots with 5-0 suture).

Vertical or Horizontal Mattress Suture

The vertical mattress suture promotes eversion and is useful where thick layers are encountered or tension exists. Two techniques may be used. The classic method first places the deep stitch and closes with the superficial stitch (Fig. 11.11). The short-hand method[22] is performed by placing the shallow stitch first, pulling up on the suture (tenting the skin), and then placing the deeper stitch. Horizontal mattress sutures also have the advantage of needing fewer knots to cover the same area.

Intracuticular Running Suture

The intracuticular running suture, utilizing a nonabsorbable suture, can be used where there is minimal skin tension. It results in minimal scarring without suture marks. Controlled tissue apposition is difficult with this method, but it is a popular technique because of the cosmetic result. The suture ends do not need to be tied but can be taped in place under slight tension (Fig. 11.12).

Three-Point Mattress Suture

The three-point or corner stitch is used to minimize the possibility of vascular necrosis of the tip of a V-shaped wound. The needle is inserted

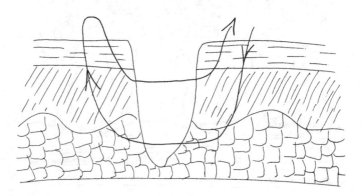

Fig. 11.11. Vertical mattress suture.

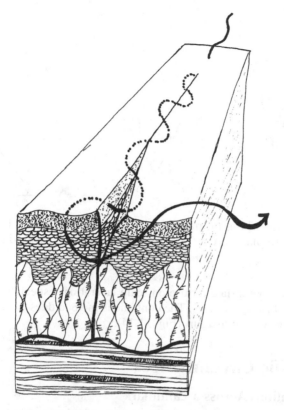

Fig. 11.12. Intracuticular running stitch.

into the skin of the wound edge on one side of the wound opposite the flap near the apex of the wound (Fig. 11.13A,B). The suture is placed at the mid-dermis level, brought across the wound, and placed transversely at the same level through the apex of the flap. It is then brought across the wound and returned at the same level on the opposite side of the V parallel to the point of entry. The suture is then tied, drawing the tip of the wound into position without compromising the blood supply (Fig. 11.13C). This method can also be used for stellate injuries where multiple tips can be approximated in purse-string fashion.

Running or Continuous Stitch

The running stitch is useful in situations where speed is important (e.g., a field emergency) because individual knots do not have to be

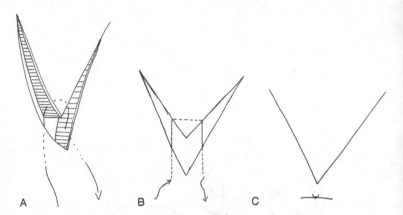

Fig. 11.13. Three-point stitch. (A) Three-dimensional view showing suture placement. (B) Schematic view. (C) Finished stitch.

tied. It is appropriate for use on scalp lacerations especially, because it is good for hemostasis. The continuous method does not allow fine control of wound margins (Fig. 11.14).

Specific Circumstances

Lacerations Across a Landmark

Lacerations that involve prominent anatomic features or landmarks, such as the vermilion border of the lip or the eyebrow, require special consideration. Commonly a laceration is closed from one end to the other, but in special situations it is advisable to place a retention stitch (a simple or vertical mattress stitch) to reapproximate the landmark border accurately. The remainder of the wound can then be closed by an appropriate method. If the retention stitch is under significant tension when the repair seems complete, it should be removed and replaced.

Beveled Lacerations

A frequently seen injury, the beveled laceration, tempts the physician to close it as it is; but the undercut flap may not heal well owing to disruption of the blood supply. The margins of the wound should be modified, as shown in Figure 11.15. The edges are squared, undermined, and closed in layers.

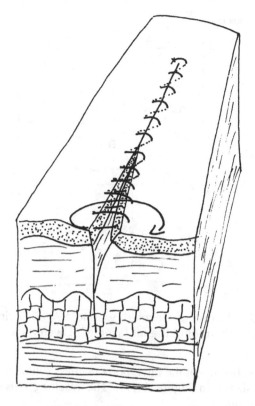

Fig. 11.14. Running stitch.

Dog Ears

Dog ear, a common problem, results from wound closure where the sides of the laceration are unequal. One side bunches up, and a mound of skin occurs. It also occurs when an elliptical wound is closed in the center, leaving excess tissue at each end. To correct the problem, the dog ear is tented up with a skin hook, and a linear incision is made along one side. The excess triangle is then grasped at the tip and a second linear incision is made (Fig. 11.16). This maneuver allows closure in a single line.

Complex Lacerations

A wound may occur with unequal sides with a hump of tissue on one side. This lump of tissue may be excised using the technique described above for removal of dog ears. The triangular defect is then closed

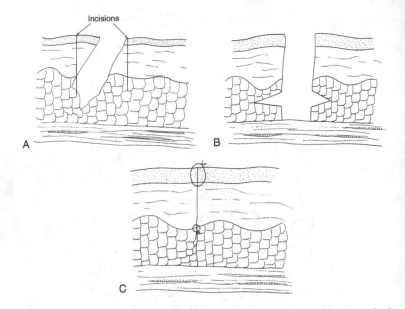

Fig. 11.15. Closure of beveled wound. (A) Squaring beveled edges. (B) Undermining the fat layer. (C) Layered closure.

using a modification of the three-point mattress suture, the four-point technique shown in Figure 11.17. The resulting closure forms a T-shaped repair.

Finger Injuries

Amputated Fingertip

If the area of the fingertip amputation is less than 1 cm², the wound can be handled by careful cleansing, proper dressings, and subsequent healing by secondary intention. If the wound is larger, the complexity of treatment increases. If the amputation is beveled dorsally and distally, a conservative approach without suturing or grafting usually results in good healing. An unfavorable angle requires more extensive repair.[23] Referral to a plastic or hand surgeon may be warranted.

Nail Bed Injuries

Nail bed injuries can be managed by saving the nail and reapproximating nail matrix lacerations with fine absorbable sutures. It may be necessary to remove the nail to repair an underlying nail bed tear. The

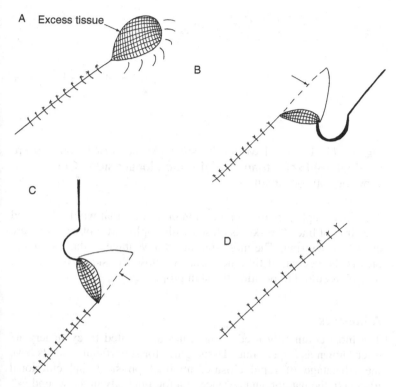

Fig. 11.16. Correction of "dog ear." (A) Excess tissue at end of repair. (B) Tenting the dog ear and first incision. (C) Pulling flap across initial incision and position of second incision. (D) Appearance of final closure.

nail may then be replaced and held in position with several sutures, allowing the nail to act as a splint.

Alternatives to Suturing

Suturing has been an effective method for closing wounds for centuries, but options for skin suturing are now available. They may even represent more cost-effective methods of wound closure.

Staples

One option is the use of skin staples, which have been used for years in the operating room as the final closure for a variety of incisions.

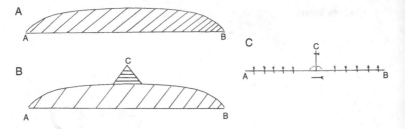

Fig. 11.17. Unequal wound closure. (A) Sides of laceration are unequal. (B) Excise triangle of tissue on longer side. (C) T-closure showing four-point suture.

Typically, staples are used on the skin in wounds that would be closed in a straight line. The skin is closed with staples after other layers are closed by suturing. The most significant advantage to the use of staples is the decreased time necessary to close the skin. An assistant may be required to position the skin properly.[24]

Adhesives

The most commonly used tissue glues are related to cyanoacrylate ester known as Super Glue. Tissue glues for superficial wounds have the advantage of rapid closure, minimal physical and emotional trauma to the patient, and absence of a foreign body in the wound.[25,26] They may also be less expensive to use than traditional methods of closure.

Histoacryl Blue, a.k.a. Dermabond, has been commercially available in Canada since 1975, and in the United States since 1998. It is a safe alternative to suturing.[27–29] Hemostasis must be achieved before applying the glue. Because some chemicals used for hemostasis such as Monsel's solution will prevent the adhesive from bonding to the skin, care must be taken to avoid skin edges. Layered closure may be accomplished using deep, absorbable sutures combined with surface adhesive. Surface sutures combined with adhesive should be avoided because the adhesive will bond to the suture material and may make removing the suture difficult. Only wounds that are under no tension are appropriate for adhesive, such as those on the face and the forearm. Even wounds such as on the foot are generally inappropriate because as soon as the patient steps on the foot, pressure is generated across the wound edges. After hemostasis and cleansing have been achieved, the wound must be approximated using gloved fingers (vinyl is preferred to latex because it also does not bond as well to the adhesive), metal instruments (preferred because metal also does not bond as tightly to the adhesive as plastic), Steri-strips, or specially manufactured closure devices for use with the adhesive. With the wound edges approximated, a layer of adhesive is applied to the top of the wound and allowed to polymerize. Two more subsequent layers should be applied and allowed to polymerize over the top of the first layer. Some other precautions: because the adhesive is a very thin, runny liquid, gravity should be utilized to keep the liquid from running into eyes, the wound itself, or other undesirable areas. If adhesive does get on the cornea in spite of appropriate precautions, it does not cause damage and may be left to come off within a few days. Other methods to control the spread of the adhesive include sponges lightly moistened with saline or use of Vaseline around the area. The patient should be instructed to keep the wound dry for 7 to 10 days because moisture weakens the bonding strength. The wound can either be left open to air, or covered with a clean bandage. Petroleum-based products should also be avoided on the adhesive because of a weakening effect.

Postrepair Management

Most wounds should be protected during the first 1 to 2 days after repair. Frequently a commercial bandage may be used; but when the wound is still oozing, a pressure dressing is applied. The initial layer is a nonstick gauze dressing available in sterile packages, such as Adaptic, Telfa, or Xeroderm. A gauze pad is then placed and held in place by roller gauze, elastic wrap, or elastic tape. Dressings are removed and the wound reexamined at 48 to 72 hours. If a drain has been placed, it should be advanced every 24 to 48 hours. If the wound is under significant tension, additional support can be achieved by using Steri-Strips or bulky supportive dressings, including splints that are commercially available or custom-made from plaster or fiberglass.

Most wounds can be left open after the first 24 to 48 hours. It is important to remove wet dressings from a repair because the skin maceration that results from them may prolong healing and increase the risk of infection. Initial epithelialization takes place during the first 24 hours, and thereafter it is permissible to wash the wound briefly. Lacerations on the scalp and face may be impractical to bandage.

Wounds should be reexamined for infection or hematoma formation after 2 to 3 days if there is any concern at the time of repair. Contaminated wounds and wounds that have been open longer than 24 hours have a greater likelihood of infection.

Timing of suture removal should be individualized, based on wound location, the mechanical stress placed on the repair, and the tension of the closure. Facial sutures should be removed within 3 to 5 days to minimize the possibility of suture tracks. Supporting the repair with Steri-Strips may decrease the likelihood of dehiscence. In skin areas that are not highly mobile (e.g., the back or extremities) sutures are left in place for 7 to 10 days. On fingers, palms, soles, and over joints, the sutures remain in place at least 10 to 14 days and sometimes longer. Table 11.2 is a sample instruction sheet for patients.

Concurrent Therapy

Preventing infection is an important aspect of laceration treatment. Puncture wounds and bites usually should not be closed because the risk of infection negates the advantage of closure. Dog bites can usually be safely closed, however. Sometimes a gaping puncture wound on the face requires closure for cosmetic reasons despite the risk of infection.

Antibiotic Usage

Antibiotic prophylaxis is probably not helpful in most circumstances unless given in sufficient quantity to obtain good tissue levels while

Table 11.2. **Instructions for Patients**

1. Keep wound dressings clean and dry. Protect dressings from moisture when bathing.
2. If the dressing gets wet, remove it and reapply a clean, dry dressing.
3. Remove the dressing after 2 days and reapply every 2 days unless instructed otherwise.
4. If any of the following signs appear, contact your physician or clinic immediately.
    A. Wound becomes red, warm, swollen, or tender.
    B. Wound begins to drain.
    C. Red streaks appear near the wound or up the arm or leg.
    D. Tender lumps appear in the armpit or groin.
    E. Chills or fever occur.
5. Because of your particular injury the doctor would like your wound check in _____ days.
6. Please return for removal of your stitches in _____ days.
7. You received the following vaccinations:
    A. Tetanus toxoid _____
    B. DT (diphtheria/tetanus) _____
    C. DPT (diphtheria/pertussis/tetanus) _____

the wound is still open. If extensive repair is necessary, intravenous antibiotics should be started during wound closure. Animal and human bite wounds are often treated by post-closure antibiotics. The efficacy of this practice remains controversial, but antibiotics are often given because of the extensive contamination that occurs with bite wounds, especially those from cats. Amoxicillin-clavulanate covers the typical bacteria of bite wounds. Doxycycline and ceftriaxone are alternative medications.[29]

Tetanus Prophylaxis

Tetanus prophylaxis is a crucial part of the care of the lacerated patient; it is imperative that the immunization status of the patient be documented. Patients most likely to be inadequately immunized are the elderly, who may have never received a primary series. Table 11.3 is a summary of the guide published by the Centers for Disease Control and Prevention. Whenever passive immunity is required, human tetanus immune globulin (TIg) is preferred. The usual dose of TIg is 500 units IM. Tetanus toxoid and TIg should be given through separate needles at separate sites.[30,31]

Table 11.3. **Guide to Tetanus Prophylaxis During Routine Wound Management**

History of adsorbed tetanus toxoid (doses)	Clean, minor wounds		All other wounds[a]	
	Td[b]	TIg	Td[b]	TIg
Unknown or <3	Yes	No	Yes	Yes
≥Three[c]	No[d]	No	No[e]	No

[a]Such as, but not limited to, wounds contaminated with dirt, feces, soil, and saliva; puncture wounds; avulsions; and wounds resulting from missiles, crushing, burns, and frostbite.

[b]For children <7 years old; DPT (DT if pertussis vaccine is contraindicated) is preferred to tetanus toxoid alone. For persons ≥7 years of age Td is preferred to tetanus toxoid alone.

[c]If only three doses of *fluid* toxoid have been received, a fourth dose of toxoid, preferably an adsorbed toxoid, is given.

[d]Yes, if >10 years since last dose.

[e]Yes, if >5 years since last dose. (More frequent boosters are not needed and can accentuate side effects.)

Td = tetanus-diphtheria toxoid; TIg = tetanus immune globulin; DPT = diphtheria/pertussis/tetanus.

References

1. Brietenbach KL, Bergera JJ. Principles and techniques of primary wound closure. Prim Care 1986;13:411–31.
2. Snell G. Laceration repair. In: Pfenninger JL, Fowler GC, eds. Procedures for primary care physicians. St. Louis: Mosby, 1994;12–19.
3. Bonadio WA, Wagner V. Efficacy of TAC topical anesthetic for repair of pediatric lacerations. Am J Dis Child 1988;142:203–5.
4. Hegenbarth MA, Altieri MF, Hawk WH, Green A, Ochsenschlager DW, O'Donnell R. Comparison of topical tetracaine, adrenaline, and cocaine anesthesia with lidocaine infiltration for repair of lacerations in children. Ann Emerg Med 1990;19:63–7.
5. Matsumoto AH, Reifsnyder AC, Hartwell GD, Angle JF, Selby JB, Tegtmeyer CJ. Reducing the discomfort of lidocaine administration through pH buffering. J Vasc Interv Radiol 1994;5:171–5.
6. Bartfield JM, Ford DT, Homer PJ. Buffered versus plain lidocaine for digital nerve blocks. Ann Emerg Med 1993;22:216–19.
7. Mader TJ, Playe SJ, Garb JL. Reducing the pain of local anesthetic infiltration: warming and buffering have a synergistic effect. Ann Emerg Med 1994;23:550–4.
8. Brogan BX Jr, Giarrusso E, Hollander JE, Cassara G, Mararnga MC, Thode HC. Comparison of plain, warmed, and buffered lidocaine for anesthesia of traumatic wounds. Ann Emerg Med 1995;26:121–5.
9. Murakami CS, Odland PB, Ross BK. Buffered local anesthetics and epinephrine degradation. J Dermatol Surg Oncol 1994;20:192–5.
10. Thompson KD, Welykyj S, Massa MC. Antibacterial activity of lidocaine in combination with a bicarbonate buffer. J Dermatol Surg Oncol 1993;19:216–20.
11. Ernst AA, Marvez-Valls E, Mall G, Patterson J, Xie X, Weiss SJ. 1% lidocaine versus 0.5% diphenhydramine for local anesthesia in minor laceration repair. Ann Emerg Med 1994;23:1328–32.
12. Task Force on Sedation and Analgesia by Non-Anesthesiologists. Practical guidelines for sedation and analgesia by non-anesthesiologists. Anesthesiology 1996;84:459–71.
13. Qureshi FA, Mellis PT, McFadden MA. Efficacy of oral ketamine for providing sedation and analgesia to children requiring laceration repair. Pediatr Emerg Care 1995;11:93–7.
14. Connors K, Terndrup TE. Nasal versus oral midazolam for sedation of anxious children undergoing laceration repair. Ann Emerg Med 1994;24:1074–9.
15. Shane SA, Fuchs SM, Khine H. Efficacy of rectal midazolam for the sedation of preschool children undergoing laceration repair. Ann Emerg Med 1994;24:1065–73.
16. Schutzman SA, Burg J, Liebelt E, et al. Oral transmucosal fentanyl citrate for the premedication of children undergoing laceration repair. Ann Emerg Med 1994;24:1059–64.
17. Clinical considerations in the use of fentanyl Oralet. North Chicago, IL: Abbott Laboratories, 1995;1–16.
18. Gamis AS, Knapp JF, Glenski JA. Nitrous oxide analgesia in a pediatric emergency department. Ann Emerg Med 1989;18:177–81.

19. Moy RL, Lee A, Zolka A. Commonly used suture materials in skin surgery. Am Fam Physician 1991;44:2123–8.
20. Epperson WJ. Suture selection. In: Pfenninger JL, Fowler GC, eds. Procedures for primary care physicians. St. Louis: Mosby, 1994;3–6.
21. Moy RL, Waldman B, Hein DW. A review of sutures and suturing techniques. J Dermatol Surg Oncol 1992;18:785–95.
22. Jones JS, Gartner M, Drew G, Pack S. The shorthand vertical mattress stitch: evaluation of a new suture technique. Am J Emerg Med 1993;11: 483–5.
23. Ditmars DM Jr. Finger tip and nail bed injuries. Occup Med 1989;4: 449–61.
24. Edlich RF, Thacker JG, Silloway RF, Morgan RF, Rodeheaver GT. Scientific basis of skin staple closure. In: Haval Mutaz B, ed. Advances in plastic and reconstructive surgery. Chicago: Year Book, 1986;233–71.
25. Osmond MH, Klassen TP, Quinn JV. Economic comparison of a tissue adhesive and suturing in the repair of pediatric facial lacerations. J Pediatr 1995;126(6):892–5.
26. Quinn JV, Drzewiecki A, Li MM, et al. A randomized, controlled trial comparing tissue adhesive with suturing in the repair of pediatric facial lacerations. Ann Emerg Med 1993;22:1130–5.
27. Applebaum JS, Zalut T, Applebaum D. The use of tissue adhesive for traumatic laceration repair in the emergency department. Ann Emerg Med 1993;22:1190–2.
28. Fisher AA. Reactions to cyanoacrylate adhesives: "instant glue." Cutis 1995:18–22,46,58.
29. Lewis KT, Stiles M. Management of cat and dog bites. Am Fam Physician 1995;52:479–85.
30. Centers for Disease Control. Tetanus prophylaxis during routine wound management. MMWR 1991;40(RR-10):1–28.
31. Richardson JP, Knight AL. The management and prevention of tetanus. J Emerg Med 1993;11:737–42.

12
Selected Injuries

Allan V. Abbott

Unintentional injuries remain the fifth leading cause of death in the United States. Table 12.1 lists these deaths according to cause and frequency.[1]

Near-Drowning

Drowning is the third leading cause of accidental death in the United States, accounting for about 4000 deaths annually. *Near-drowning* is defined as survival after an episode of suffocation and cerebral hypoxia in a liquid medium, whereas *submersion injury* (*drowning*) is death within 24 hours of such an episode. *Secondary drowning* is death from complications that occur more than 24 hours after the submersion. *Immersion syndrome* is sudden death after contact with cold water.[2]

Most near-drownings and drownings occur among inadequately supervised children younger than 4 years of age in swimming pools, ocean surf, bathtubs, or hot tubs. In small children, drowning is more common than toxic ingestions and firearm injuries. Boys and young men between the ages of 15 and 24 and the elderly over age 75, especially if unable to swim, are also at risk because of alcohol or drug use while swimming, infirmity, or associated trauma or seizures.

Clinical Presentation

The usual submerged drowning victim at first holds his or her breath and becomes anoxic and panics, then swallows or gasps and aspirates water, loses consciousness, and dies in cardiac arrest. Approximately 10% of victims have acute laryngospasm that results in dry drowning,

Table 12.1. **Deaths Due to Unintentional Injuries—United States, 1999**[1]

Type of injury	Deaths per year
All unintentional injuries	96,900
Motor vehicle accidents	41,300
Falls	17,100
Drowning	4,000
Suffocation by ingested object	3,200
Fires and burns	3,100
Firearms	700
Poisoning by gas and vapors	500
All other	16,500

because there is no aspiration of water into the lungs and death typically occurs owing to profound obstructive asphyxia.[2]

The duration of hypoxia that can be tolerated depends on the individual's age and health, the water temperature, and the promptness and effectiveness of the resuscitation. Young victims usually recover if the submersion is less than 3 minutes, or up to 10 minutes if the water is cold (0°–15°C) (32°–59°F). Survival has been reported after 15 to 20 minutes of submersion and up to 40 minutes in cold water.[3]

With near-drowning the clinical presentation depends on the stage at which the drowning sequence was interrupted. Aspiration of water leads to varying degrees of pulmonary edema and can result in adult respiratory distress syndrome as late as 72 hours after the near-drowning. There may be shortness of breath, rales, rhonchi, or wheezing. Chest radiographs may initially show pulmonary edema or appear misleadingly normal. Severe pulmonary edema can develop slowly in a patient who initially has no pulmonary signs or symptoms. Hypothermia due to submersion in cold water often leads to bradycardia or atrial fibrillation. Hypoxia leads to cerebral damage with subsequent cerebral edema. Internal injuries should be suspected with falls into the water and boating accidents; cervical spine and head injuries are particularly common. Severe acidosis and electrolyte disturbances can occur. Subsequent intravascular hemolysis, disseminated intravascular coagulation, and renal failure are uncommon but possible.

Management
Immediate Management
Aggressive emergency resuscitation is the most important factor influencing outcome.[4] Airway protection and respiratory support should begin immediately, even before removal from the water. Advanced

cardiopulmonary life support (ACLS) is begun immediately as indicated by the circulatory status and cardiac rhythm. Maneuvers to promote postural drainage, such as that advocated by Heimlich et al,[5] are controversial, with most experts discouraging their use because of interruption of cardiopulmonary resuscitation, loss of airway control, aspiration, and aggravation of possible cervical spine injuries.[6] Oxygen at 100% is administered to all near-drowning victims as soon it is available.

Hospital Management

The initial appearance of near-drowning patients who are conscious may be deceptively normal. Therefore, virtually all near-drowning patients should be admitted for observation, oxygen, and supportive care. If they remain asymptomatic and if chest films and arterial blood gas assays remain normal, they may be discharged after 8 hours, or after 24 hours if there was any aspiration. A large-bore intravenous line should be positioned. The rectal temperature is measured; and if the patient is hypothermic ($<35°C$, $<95°F$), rewarming is begun. Most serious cases are reflected in lactic acidosis and electrolyte disturbances, and treatment is guided by monitoring the arterial blood gases and serum electrolytes.

Patients are monitored for respiratory and central nervous system (CNS) function. Indications for endotracheal intubation in hospitalized patients include (1) protection of the airway in nearly comatose patients, (2) neurologic deterioration, (3) copious secretions or gross aspiration of particulate matter, and (4) inability to maintain a PaO_2 of 60 to 90 mm Hg. Positive end-expiratory pressure (PEEP) is helpful with a pulmonary injury to recruit gas exchange in spaces and to prevent terminal airway closure. A nasogastric tube is placed to remove excess swallowed water and air.

Bronchospasm can be managed with β-adrenergic aerosols. Early therapeutic bronchoscopy should be considered if particulate matter such as vomitus or mud have been aspirated. Most centers currently employ supportive care and do not use prophylactic antibiotics, barbiturates, steroids, hypothermia, hyperventilation, intracranial pressure monitoring, or neuromuscular blockade routinely.[2]

Survival after near-drowning and cerebral anoxia can be predicted by neurological examination 24 hours after the drowning incident. The absence of spontaneous, purposeful movements and normal brainstem function after 24 hours suggests severe neurologic deficits or death. Satisfactory recovery can be expected in presence of spontaneous, purposeful movements and normal brainstem function.[6]

Children who are involved in bathtub near-drownings may have suffered from abuse or neglect. In these cases the medical evaluation should include a social work consultation and a search for accompanying injuries.[7]

Prevention

Physicians should counsel parents that most drownings of small children can be prevented if pools and hot tubs are surrounded by a fence of at least 55 inches in height with locked or self-closing, self-latching gates, if pool safety covers are in place, and if house door-opening alarms are used.[3]

Adults should provide immediate supervision at all times when children have access to pools. Children should always wear life jackets while in boats. Adults should be trained in basic cardiopulmonary resuscitation. Also, swimming must be avoided while under the influence of alcohol or psychoactive drugs.

Barotrauma

Barotrauma—injury caused by barometric pressure changes—usually results from diving under water, ascending into the atmosphere, or mechanical respiratory support. As one ascends into the atmosphere, the atmospheric pressure decreases gradually; at 5500 m (18,000 feet) it reaches a pressure of about one half that at sea level. In contrast, when one descends into water, the pressure of the water increases more rapidly, with a doubling of pressure every 10 m (33 feet) below the surface. Barotrauma resulting from changes in atmospheric pressure occurs commonly to the ear and sinuses. Among divers, barotrauma results in ear and sinus injuries, decompression sickness, and air embolism. Pulmonary barotrauma can result from diving or mechanical ventilation.

Ear and Sinus Barotrauma

Barotrauma can affect the external ear canal, middle ear, inner ear, and sinuses. It is sometimes referred to as the "squeeze" when the ambient pressures are greater than the pressures within the body cavities; it is called "reverse squeeze" under the opposite conditions.

External Barotitis

Ear canal squeeze occurs when divers descend with ear canals plugged with earplugs or cerumen. The diver experiences pain and bloody drainage as the pressure in the middle ear exceeds that within the canal. On examination of the tympanic membrane, petechiae, hemorrhagic blebs, and rupture may be seen.[8]

Barotitis Media

Barotitis media is the most common ear injury resulting from pressure. The eustachian tube provides the only route for air to enter or exit the middle ear. The normally functioning eustachian tube acts as a one-way valve, allowing excess pressures to vent passively from the middle ear while allowing air to enter only with active swallowing, yawning, or autoinflation (the patient holds nose and mouth shut, blows to puff cheeks, and swallows with cheeks puffed).[8] When eustachian tube function is impaired by mucosal inflammation due to upper respiratory infection (URI), allergy, or trauma, the active movement of air into the inner ear is usually impaired first, with passive venting being impaired later in more severe cases. Thus a person with a URI flying in an airplane usually finds that ear pressures adjust on ascent, but pain increases during descent if swallowing or autoinflation maneuvers fail to "pop" the ears. Commercial airliners maintain cabin pressure equal to about 6000 to 8000 feet, so severe middle ear barotrauma is unlikely.

Divers who do not achieve middle ear pressure equalization experience pain on descent. Inward bulging to the tympanic membrane, hemorrhage, and edema develop, with rupture of the tympanic membrane if descent continues.[8]

Inner Ear Barotrauma

If pressure is great enough, the oval or round window can rupture, with a sudden onset of sensorineural hearing loss, severe vertigo, tinnitus, nystagmus, and fullness in the affected ear.[9,10]

Sinus Barotrauma

The frontal and maxillary sinuses may be "squeezed" when mucosal inflammation due to URI or other condition blocks the sinus ostia. It usually occurs in divers during descent, resulting in pain and epistaxis from the area of the sinus.[9]

Management

When barotitis involves a ruptured tympanic membrane, treatment includes keeping the ear dry, giving analgesics as needed, and prohibiting swimming or flying until the tympanic membrane heals spontaneously. Decongestants and antihistamines are usually recommended. Antibiotics have been suggested but are of uncertain value. Patients should not dive or fly until they have movement of the tympanic membrane on autoinflation during otoscope examination by the physician. Patients with inner ear barotrauma should be referred to an otolaryngologist. Sinus barotrauma can be treated with decongestant nasal sprays, such as phenylephrine 0.5% (Neo-Synephrine), and oral decongestants, such as pseudoephedrine (Sudafed), which shrink the nasal mucosa to help open and drain the affected sinuses.[9] Patients with recurrent sinus barotrauma or sinus barotraumas that is resistant to medical treatment should be referred to an otolaryngologist.[11]

Decompression Sickness/Pulmonary Barotrauma

Decompression sickness ("the bends") most often occurs after divers descend and remain deeper than 10 m (33 feet). As divers increase underwater depth time, nitrogen gradually dissolves in the blood and tissues. If ascent is rapid, this nitrogen can become insoluble, forming bubbles in the bloodstream and the tissues. Decompression sickness usually manifests immediately or shortly after the dive but may occur as long as 12 hours later. Most commonly, the victim experiences steady or throbbing pain in the shoulders or elbows with some relief on "bending" the affected joint. The skin may become pruritic, with rashes and purplish mottling. Cerebral effects include headache, fatigue, inappropriate behavior, seizures, hemiplegia, and visual disturbances. Pulmonary effects include substernal pain, cough, and dyspnea.[10,12]

Pulmonary barotrauma is a risk during SCUBA diving and mechanical ventilation, especially when peak airway pressures are more than 70 cm H_2O. A scuba diver breathing compressed air who ascends from depth without exhaling runs a risk of pulmonary trauma as a result of overdistention of the lungs. Overinflated alveoli can rupture and allow air to escape into the interstitium, pleural cavity, or pulmonary vessels. Slow leakage from alveoli may produce subcutaneous or mediastinal emphysema. Subcutaneous emphysema may present as neck fullness and crepitance, dysphagia, and change in voice quality. Mediastinal emphysema may present with chest pain and dyspnea. Pneumothorax occurs in as many as 15% of patients on mechanical ventilators and is difficult to recognize on portable chest radiographs.[13]

If air enters the pulmonary vessels, the symptoms of air embolism are immediate as bubbles disseminate throughout the circulation. The CNS is most frequently affected, with neurological manifestations consistent with acute stroke. Unconsciousness, stupor, focal paralysis, sensory loss, blindness, and aphasia may be seen. Acute coronary occlusion and cardiac arrest can occur.

Treatment

Immediate recompression therapy in a compression chamber is essential for both decompression sickness and air embolization. Family physicians should know the location of the nearest recompression chamber. Until recompression is possible, the patient should remain in a horizontal position breathing oxygen with monitoring of respiratory and circulatory status, and should receive oral or isotonic intravenous fluids. The most common treatment error is failure to recompress mild or questionable cases. Dramatic recoveries from decompression sickness have occurred even after recompression was delayed for 1 week.[14] Pneumothorax is treated with a chest tube. Subcutaneous and mediastinal emphysema can be treated symptomatically unless the emphysema hinders breathing or the circulation.[10]

Prevention

To prevent barotitis, scuba divers and individuals flying in aircraft should have normally functioning eustachian tubes and be able to "clear their ears" by swallowing, yawning, or performing an autoinflation maneuver. The physician can confirm this functioning by observing each tympanic membrane with an otoscope while the patient performs an autoinflation maneuver. Each tympanic membrane visibly moves or "pops" as air enters the middle ear through the eustachian tube. Individuals with a URI who must fly should be advised to use oral decongestants before flying and a decongestant nasal spray before descent to help avoid the mild but painful middle ear barotrauma on descent. Scuba divers undergo thorough training in the prevention of all types of barotrauma as part of their scuba certification. Individuals who dive without this training are at great risk for barotrauma. Pressure-targeted ventilation that limits peak ventilator pressures to 35 cm H_2O or less can help prevent barotrauma due to mechanical ventilation.[13]

Burns

Burns are the fifth leading cause of accidental deaths, with 3100 related deaths in the United States annually.[1] Of all age groups, children have the highest incidence of burn injuries: more than half occur in preschoolers, with most resulting from hot liquids, especially hot tap water from heaters set above 54°C (129°F).[15]

Most burned patients have minor injuries that can be adequately treated on an outpatient basis. Family physicians must be able to recognize and initiate emergency care for more severe burns and inhalation injuries that require hospitalization. Severe burns can cause rapid derangements of fluids and electrolytes and can lead to sepsis. For these reasons and for the prevention management of cosmetic and functional sequelae, surgical consultation is often required.

Pathophysiology

Management of burn injuries requires an understanding of the etiology and pathophysiology of the injury. In addition to the depth and extent of the burn, several special conditions may warrant hospitalization.

The skin normally prevents fluid loss, regulates heat, and protects against infection. As skin is burned it undergoes coagulation necrosis, with cell death and loss of vascularity. Next to the dead tissues is a layer of injured cells in which the circulation is impaired. There is increased capillary permeability and rapid edema development with rapid loss of fluid and heat. This injured tissue can be damaged further by improper care, which may allow drying, trauma, or infection. Gram-positive and, in a few days, gram-negative bacteria grow rapidly on the burned surface.

Partial-thickness burns leak and sequester serous exudate, which forms a yellow, sticky eschar. During healing, scarring and contractures occur wherever the dermis is devitalized.[16]

Causes

The severity of the burn is determined by the type of burning agent, the temperature, and the duration of exposure. Temperatures less than 45°C (113°F) rarely cause cell damage, yet temperatures of 50°C (122°F) can cause burns depending on the duration of exposure. Brief flash burns and scalds tend to cause relatively superficial injury, yet flash burns can be partial-thickness burns and scalds can be full-thickness burns. Burns from flames and from adherent substances cause deeper burns. Electrical injuries may appear to be minor, yet deep tissue damage may become evident in several days, often manifesting as red urine caused by the release of myoglobin from damaged muscle. The skin of elderly patients and the very young is thin and subject to greater injury.[17]

Classification

Treatment and hospitalization decisions depend on classification of burns according to the extent of the skin burned and the depth and location of the burn. The total area of the burn can be approximated in adults using the "rule of nines," although this surface area rule varies in the young age group (Fig. 12.1).[18] Small burns can be compared to the size of the patient's hand, which is about 1% of the total skin area.

Burns are traditionally classified according to depth as first, second, or third degree; however, these terms are being replaced by superficial, superficial partial-thickness, deep partial-thickness, and full-thickness. Burn depth is rarely uniform and may be difficult to determine initially and require reevaluation after a few days.[19]

Superficial Burns (First Degree)

Superficial burns involve only the superficial epidermis, appear erythematous, and blanch with pressure. Mild sunburn is an example

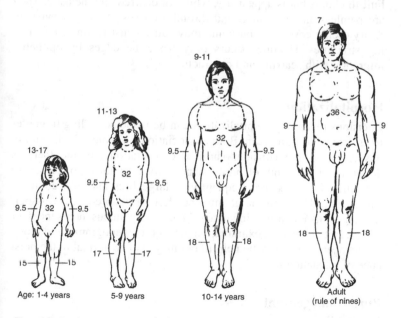

Fig. 12.1. Assessment of the percent of the total surface area. (Lund CC, Browder NC. The estimate of areas of burns. Surg Gynecol Obstet 1944;79:352–8.)

with uneventful healing and some delayed peeling. The protective functions of the skin are maintained.

Superficial and Deep Partial-Thickness Burns (Second Degree)

Superficial partial-thickness burns spare the deeper dermis components, including hair follicles and the sweat and sebaceous glands, and are either superficial or deep. These burns form bullae and are red, painful, and weeping. They blanch with pressure, and the superficial skin is sometimes wiped away. These burns heal in about 2 to 3 weeks with little or no scarring. Deep partial-thickness burns are mottled with red elements (dermal vessels) or are waxy-white and dry and do not blanch with pressure. They may be nearly painless, with sensation only to pressure. These burns may take a month or more to heal and usually form scars. They may progress to full-thickness burns if not properly treated and take 3 weeks or more to heal.

Full-Thickness Burns (Third Degree)

Full-thickness burns appear dry, white, or charred and inelastic. They are painless and avascular, and thrombosed vessels may be visible. A dry eschar covers the burn and may cause constriction of underlying structures. Healing occurs only from the edges by epithelial migration with scarring and contracture.[15]

Hospitalization

Decisions regarding hospitalization can be made according to guidelines from the American Burn Association[20] (Table 12.2). Family physicians should consider surgical consultation anytime there is doubt about the depth of burns or need for hospitalization. Because inhalation injury occurs frequently in large fires and is a common cause of death, the physician must be alert for the presence of associated signs: facial burns, singed nasal hair, sooty mucus, hoarseness, or cough. Initial physical examination, chest roentgenograms, and blood gas measurements may be helpful but may also be normal in the presence of inhalation injury.

Burn Management

Severe Burns

Immediately after the burn, the victim's clothing and any hot substances remaining in contact with the skin are removed, and the victim

Table 12.2. **Burns Requiring Hospitalization**[20]

Moderate burns (require hospitalization)

Partial-thickness burns on 15–25% of total body surface area (2–10% in children or elderly)

Full-thickness burns on 2–10% of body surface

Suspected inhalation injury

Suspected high-voltage (200 volts) electrical burns (may appear mild initially)

Circumferential burn (decompressive escharotomy may be needed)

Major burns (consider referral to burn center)

Partial-thickness burns on >25% body surface (>20% in children or elderly)

Full-thickness burns on >10% of body

Burns with inhalation injury, major trauma, or other poor risk condition such as diabetes or immunodeficiency that increase risk of infection

High-voltage (200 volts) electrical burns (may appear mild initially)

All but minimal burns to face, eyes, feet, hands, perineum, or genitalia where cosmetic or functional impairment is likely

Burns from caustic chemicals such as hydrofluoric acid (may appear mild initially)

---

is covered with a dry, sterile sheet. Copious irrigation with water is indicated for chemical injuries. Cool compresses (not ice) can be used to relieve the pain of small burns but can cause hypothermia if used for large burns. Breathing is assessed immediately and oxygen administered if there is any distress or suspicion of carbon monoxide inhalation.[21]

Airway. Early endotracheal intubation is warranted at the first indication of inhalation injury. All patients with inhalation injury should be placed on humidified oxygen. Steroids are warranted only in the presence of bronchospasm. Bronchoscopy can confirm large airway injury, and lung scans can detect small airway damage.

Fluids. Patients with burns of more than 15% to 20% of the surface area require intravenous fluid replacement. Lactated Ringer's solution at a rate of 4 mL/kg per percent of burned area during the first 24 hours is the most common fluid replacement regimen used in the United States, with half of this amount given during the first 8 hours after the burn. Many other fluid regimens have been used, but all must be administered with close monitoring of renal output and cardiovascular status.

Pain Management. Narcotics and benzodiazepines are used initially for relief of pain and anxiety *with caution* because they can exacerbate the hypotension that may follow a major burn. Immediate administration of narcotics may also interfere with evaluation of other associated trauma. After intravenous fluids have been administered and fluid status has stabilized, narcotic doses can be increased. Inhaled or intravenous anesthesia may be needed for the severe pain of early dressing changes.[22]

Consultation. Consultation with a surgical burn specialist is appropriate for all severe burns, small burns that are deep partial-thickness or deeper, and those located on the face, eyes, ears, or neck or in areas of critical function including the hands, elbows, popliteal fossae, or feet. Major complications including sepsis and hypermetabolism, and subsequent major burn management is best handled in major burn centers.[23]

Minor Burns

Minor burns, those not requiring hospitalization, are by far the most common type of burn managed by the family physician. Partial-thickness burns contain portions of epithelium that must be protected from further damage so epithelialization can occur.

Local Care. For all burns, the clothing and any hot or caustic materials are removed immediately; and cool saline-soaked gauze is applied. The ideal temperature for those compresses is 12°C (54°F), which avoids hypothermia while relieving pain and increasing circulation for up to 3 hours after the burn. Burns are cleaned with saline or mild soapy water; the use of chlorhexidine gluconate (Hibiclens) or half-strength povidone-iodine (Betadine) is now discouraged because these agents may inhibit healing. Cytotoxic cleansing agents such as hydrogen peroxide should be avoided. Necrotic skin is carefully removed using aseptic technique; whirlpool debridement is often well tolerated by patients. The yellow eschar of partial-thickness burns should not be removed initially. Blisters may be left intact but are removed if they appear to contain cloudy fluid, if broken, or if they cover possible full-thickness burns.

Topical chemoprophylaxis is used for all but superficial burns to prevent infection. Silver sulfadiazine (Silvadene) cream, classically the most commonly used topical agent, is applied to the burn in a thickness of about 1 to 2 mm and is then covered with a loose-fitting dressing such as soft gauze. Silver sulfadiazine should not be used on the face, on patients with sulfonamide sensitivity, or in pregnant patients. Bacitracin (Baciguent) ointment is a good alternative. Systemic antibiotics are used only with a proved burn infection. Oral nonsteroidal antiinflammatory drugs, acetaminophen with codeine, and rarely narcotics, can be given for pain.[15]

An alternative to topical chemoprophylaxis and dressing changes for superficial partial-thickness burns (not deeper burns) is the use of synthetic dressings such as Duoderm, Opsite, or Biobrane.[24] These expensive dressings are applied to fresh, clean, moist burns and are left in place until the burn heals or until the dressing separates in about 1 to 2 weeks. In many cases these dressings are easy to use, promote fast healing, decrease infection, do not limit activity, reduce pain, and are acceptable to the patient overall. Immunity to tetanus should be ensured, as burns are readily subject to tetanus infections.[25] (See Table 11.3.)

Follow-Up Care. Patients should bathe daily and gently wash off completely and reapply the silver sulfadiazine. Dressings should remain intact under any circumstances where the burns might become dirty but may be removed at home when the burns can be protected. The physician should recheck partial-thickness burns daily, and patients should be alert to signs of impaired circulation caused by a tight dressing and to signs of infection such as chills or fever. The physician should remain alert for hypertrophic scarring and contractures and refer these patients to a burn specialist. Depending upon depth, 6 to 24 months may be required for complete healing; during this period the healing skin should be protected from sun exposure and lubricated with moisturizing cream.[26]

Sunburn

Superficial burns resulting from sunburn are common in fair-skinned individuals and frequently come to the attention of the family physician. The skin appears red, blanches with light pressure, and is tender and painful. Skin lubricants such as Eucerin may improve comfort. The use of topical anesthetic sprays should be limited because they may sensitize the skin to the anesthetics. Topical steroids have little effect; but with extensive sunburns, constitutional symptoms may be improved with oral prednisone at a daily dose of 20 mg for 2 to 3 days.

Prevention

Prevention of most burns takes place in the home by the family. Water heaters should be set to a temperature below 51°C (124°F) to avoid scalds. Smoke detectors should be installed and checked regularly. Electrical outlets should be covered to protect children from electrical injury, and chemicals and caustic agents must be stored away from the reach of children. In the kitchen, hot pot handles should be turned away from children, and all foods should be temperature-tested before being offered to children. Oily rags must be discarded and flammables stored properly. Finally, sunscreens should be used to prevent sunburn, and sun exposure should be avoided between 10 A.M. and 4 P.M.

As many as one in five burns of young children are the result of abusive acts, so abuse must be considered when a child has more than two burn sites, burns at various stages of healing, and burns that follow a particular pattern (e.g., "stocking-glove" distribution).[27] When abuse is suspected, evaluation of previous medical records, checking with protective services, and hospital admission should be considered.

Aspirated or Swallowed Foreign Body

Pathophysiology

More deaths in the United States result from suffocation by foreign bodies than from burns or from firearms accidents. Children younger than 3 years of age have a natural tendency to place objects in their mouths, putting them at high risk of choking injury. In children younger than 1 year, asphyxiation is an important cause of unintentional death. The foreign bodies most often aspirated are food, including nuts, vegetable or fruit pieces, seeds, and popcorn. Small items such as pen caps, beads, or crayons may be aspirated by small children. Balloons pose a high risk for aspiration and asphyxiation to children of any age. Items that may become lodged in the cricopharyngeus or esophagus include coins, pieces of food, pieces of toys or hardware, batteries, glass, chicken bones, etc.[28]

Large objects in the esophagus can cause airway obstruction. The gastrointestinal (GI) tract can become obstructed or perforated; mediastinitis, cardiac tamponade, paraesophageal abscess, or aortotracheoesophageal fistula can occur. Perforation may be the result of direct mechanical erosion (bones), or chemical corrosion (button batteries).[29]

Most pediatric obstructions occur in the proximal esophagus, and most obstructions in adults occur at the distal esophagus in those with a history of esophageal disease. Most swallowed foreign bodies that pass through the esophagus continue through the entire GI tract without difficulty, but 10% to 20% require some intervention and about 1% require surgery. Objects larger than 3 to 5 cm may have difficulty passing the duodenal loop in the region of the ligament of Treitz.

Clinical Manifestations

The most frequent symptom of aspirated foreign body is a sudden onset of choking and intractable cough with or without vomiting. Other presenting symptoms may be cough, fever, breathlessness, and wheezing. Some patients will be asymptomatic and many, especially older adults, are misdiagnosed as having other pulmonary diseases. On chest radiograph a pneumonic patch or atelectasis may be present in adults, and air trapping is more common in children. Older adults predisposed to aspiration include those with stroke or other central nervous system disease or major underlying lung disease.[30]

A swallowed foreign body can be painful and can provoke great anxiety. Foreign bodies in the esophagus usually cause dysphagia, especially with solid foods, and occasionally dyspnea due to compression of the larynx. Patients may be unable to swallow their own secretions. The initial period may be symptom-free, with symptoms of esophageal obstruction developing later as the result of edema and inflammation. Increasing pain, fever, and shock suggest perforation.[31]

Management

When an aspirated foreign body is suspected or diagnosed on chest radiograph, bronchoscopy is indicated. Success of foreign body removal by bronchoscopy depends on the experience of the bronchoscopist.

Because most ingested foreign bodies pass without problems, evaluation and treatment are often expectant. When patients complain of a sticking sensation in their throat (as is often the case when a fish bone is swallowed), direct or indirect laryngoscopy permits direct visualization and removal with forceps. Esophagogastroscopy is preferred for removal of most foreign bodies lodged in the esophagus or stomach. Radiopaque foreign bodies can be easily diagnosed with standard radiographs of the neck, chest, or abdomen. An esophagram can be used to locate nonopaque objects. The physical examination is repeated to detect signs of obstruction or early peritonitis with perforation. The progress of the object through the GI tract can be monitored with repeat abdominal films. If a foreign body remains in one position distal to the pylorus for longer than 5 days, surgical removal should be considered.

Food Impaction

The typical patient with an esophageal food impaction is elderly, usually a denture wearer. The history is usually that the patient swallowed a bolus of meat and feels that it is caught "halfway down." Complete occlusion is evident when the patient cannot swallow water and regurgitates. The airway is usually uninvolved, and the patient speaks and breathes without difficulty. Endoscopic removal is preferred. The use of proteolytic enzymes, such as aqueous solution of papain (e.g., Adolph's meat tenderizer) is not recommended owing to the risk of perforation. When endoscopy is not available, intravenous glucagon (1.0 mg) has been suggested to relax the esophageal smooth muscle. If the food bolus has not passed in 20 minutes, an additional 2.0 mg is given intravenously. An esophagram should be obtained to ensure passage of the impaction.

Coin Ingestion

Half of the children with coins lodged in their esophagus are asymptomatic; therefore, radiographs are obtained for all children suspected of swallowing coins. Endoscopy is the preferred and safest method of coin removal. If endoscopy is not available, a Foley catheter can be passed down the esophagus beyond the object. The balloon is then inflated, and as the catheter is slowly withdrawn the coin is withdrawn with it. There is a high incidence of aspiration with this technique in small children younger than 5 years of age. Coins have been observed to remain in the stomach for 2 to 3 months before spontaneous passage.[32]

Battery Ingestion

Most batteries pass uneventfully through the GI tract within 48 to 72 hours. However, a button battery lodged in the esophagus is an emergency. These batteries contain 45% potassium hydroxide, which is erosive to the esophagus and especially hazardous. Button batteries should be removed endoscopically from the esophagus or if they remain in the stomach longer than 24 hours.[29]

Ingestion of Sharp Objects

Children who have swallowed a sharp object yet are asymptomatic can be managed on an expectant basis.[31] Progression of the sharp object should be documented by serial radiographs. If it is not seen to progress past the stomach and perforation is suspected, a water-soluble contrast radiograph is obtained. Perforation requires prompt surgical intervention. Close observation or hospitalization is recommended for children who have swallowed open safety pins or long, sharp objects such as sewing needles.

Prevention

Young children should not have access to small objects such as toys with small detachable parts, coins, pins, and the like. Children younger than 3 years should not be given food in forms that could be aspirated; nuts, popcorn, vegetable chunks, and so on should be avoided. Care should be taken to avoid aspiration when feeding older adults who have stroke or other serious debilitating disease. If metered dose inhalers are carried in bags or pockets without their safety caps on, foreign bodies may enter their mechanism and be expelled forcefully into the bronchial tree. The ensuing symptoms are often difficult to distinguish from those of an acute attack of asthma.

Fishhook Removal

There are four basic strategies for removing a barbed fishhook when it has accidentally penetrated a person's skin. Sterile technique, local cleansing, and local anesthesia are appropriate with all the techniques. Fishhook injuries are tetanus prone, and antibiotics should be given when the wound is particularly dirty or when infection is already evident. Fishhook injuries to the eye or orbit should be referred to an ophthalmologist.[33]

Simple Retrograde Pull

If the hook has a small barb or is not embedded deeply, the hook can be held close to the skin with a needle holder or hemostat and withdrawn along its entry path (Fig. 12.2A). A small 1- to 2-mm incision may be needed to help the barb pass through the dermis.

String-Yank Technique

This technique (Fig. 12.2B) does not involve any incisions or surgical equipment and may be tried in the field. A strong suture or fishing line is passed around the bend of the hook, and both ends are held together with one hand while the hook is stabilized and gently depressed against the skin with the other. A sharp pull is applied to the suture in the direction parallel to the shank of the hook.

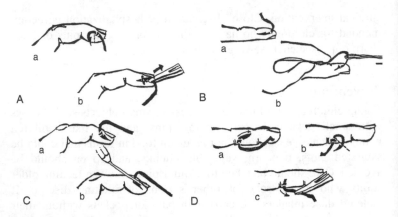

Fig. 12.2. Fishhook removal. (A) Simple retrograde pull. (B) String-yank technique. (C) Needle-cover technique. (D) Push and cut technique.

Needle-Cover Technique

The needle-cover technique (Fig. 12.2C) is often useful when the barb is large. The hook is held in a needle holder or hemostat, and a 16- or 18-gauge hypodermic needle is introduced through the entry wound and advanced along the hook's bend until the barb can be sheathed within the lumen of the needle. The hook and needle are then gently withdrawn together. It is my experience that, with practice, this technique is usually successful.

Advance and Cut Technique

This method is nearly always successful but causes additional trauma to the surrounding tissue (Fig. 12.2D). The middle of the shank is firmly grasped with a needle holder and the hook tip is advanced out through the skin. The exposed point of the hook is removed with wire cutters, and the hook shank is withdrawn from the wound in a retrograde manner.

References

1. Injury Facts, 2000 edition. Itasca, IL: National Safety Council, 2000.
2. Ramesh CS. Near drowning. Crit Care Clin 1999;15:281–96.
3. Levin DL, Morriss FC, Toro LO, Brink LW, Turner GR. Drowning and near-drowning. Pediatr Clin North Am 1993;40:321–6.

4. Christensen DW, Jansen P, Perkin RM. Outcome and acute care hospital costs after warm water near drowning in children. Pediatrics 1997;99: 715–21.

5. Heimlich H, Hoffman K, Canestri F. Food choking and drowning deaths prevented by external subdiaphragmatic compression. Ann Thorac Surg 1975;20:188–95.

6. Bratton SL, Jardine DS, Morray JP. Serial neurologic examinations after near-drowning and outcome. Arch Pediatr Adolesc Med 1994;148:167–70.

7. Lavelle JM, Shaw KN, Seidl T, Ludwig S. Ten-year review of pediatric near-drownings: evaluation for child abuse and ne-glect. Ann Emerg Med 1995;25:344–8.

8. James JR. Dysbarism: the medical problems from high and low atmospheric pressure. J R Coll Physicians Lond 1993;27:367–74.

9. Jerrard DA. Diving medicine. Emerg Med Clin North Am 1992; 10: 329–38.

10. Moon RE. Treatment of diving emergencies. Crit Care Clin 1999;15: 429–49.

11. Parell JG, Becker GD. Neurological consequences of scuba diving with chronic sinusitis. Laryngoscope 2000;110:1358–60.

12. Melamed Y, Shupak A, Bitterman H. Current concepts: medical problems associated with underwater diving. N Engl J Med 1992;326:30–5.

13. Marcy TW. Barotrauma: detection, recognition, and management. Chest 1993;104:578–84.

14. Boettger ML. Scuba diving emergencies: pulmonary overpressure accidents and decompression sickness. Ann Emerg Med 1983;12:563–7.

15. Feller I. Burn epidemiology: focus on youngsters and the aged. Burn Care Rehabil 1982;3:285.

16. Griglak MJ. Thermal injury. Emerg Med Clin North Am 1992;10: 369–83.

17. Carvajal HF. Burns in children and adolescents: initial management as the first step in successful rehabilitation. Pediatrician 1991;17:237–43.

18. Lund CC, Browder NC. The estimate of areas of burns. Surg Gynecol Obstet 1944;79:352–8.

19. Clark J. Burns. Br Med Bull 1999;55:885–94.

20. Joint Committee of the American Burn Association and the American College of Surgeons Committee on Trauma. Assessment and initial care of burn patients. Chicago: ACS, 1986.

21. Robertson C, Fenton O. ABC of major trauma: management of severe burns. BMJ 1990;301:282–6.

22. Henry DB, Foster RL. Burn pain management in children. Pediatr Clin North Am 2000;47:681–98.

23. Nguyen TT, Gilpin DA, Meyer NA, Herndon DN. Current treatment of severely burned patients. Ann Surg 1996;223:14–25.

24. Wyatt D, McGowan DS, Najarian MP. Comparison of a hydrocolloid dressing and silver sulfadiazine in the outpatient management of second-degree burns. J Trauma 1990;30:857–65.

25. Smith DJ. Burn wounds: infection and healing. Am J Surg 1994;167: 46S–8S.

26. Morgan ED, Scott CB, Barker J. Ambulatory management of burns. Am Fam Physician 2000;62:2016–26.
27. Rosenberg NM, Marino D. Frequency of suspected abuse/neglect in burn patients. Pediatr Emerg Care 1989;5:219–21.
28. Rimell FL, Thome A, Stoll S, et al. Characteristics of objects that cause choking in children. JAMA 1995;274:1763–6.
29. Litovitz T, Schmitz BE. Ingestion of cylindrical and button batteries, an analysis of 2382 cases. Pediatrics 1992;89:727.
30. Baharloo F, Veyckemans F, Francis C, et al. Tracheobronchial foreign bodies: presentation and management in children and adults. Chest 1999; 115:1357–62.
31. Paul RI, Jaffe DM. Sharp object ingestions in children: illustrative case and literature review. Pediatr Emerg Care 1988;4:245.
32. Caravati EM, Bennett DL, McElwee NE. Pediatric coin ingestion: a prospective study on the utility of routine roentgenograms. Am J Dis Child 1989;143:549.
33. Gammons M, Jackson S. Fishhook removal. Am Fam Physician 2001; 63:2231–6.

INDEX